LIZ EARLE'S
BEST
BIKINI DIET

BⒺXTREE

Advice to the Reader
*Before following any dietary advice contained in this book, it is
recommended that you consult your doctor if you suffer from any health
problems or special condition or are in any doubt as to its suitability.*

First published in Great Britain in 1995 by Boxtree Limited.
New edition published in Great Britain in 1996 by Boxtree Limited.
This edition published in 1997 by Boxtree an imprint of Macmillan
Publishers Ltd, 25 Eccleston Place, London, SW1W 9NF and Basingstoke.

The right of Liz Earle to be identified as Author of this Work has
been asserted by her in accordance with the Copyright, Designs
and Patents Act 1988

10 9 8 7 6 5 4 3 2 1

ISBN: 0 7522 2195 7

Text design by Blackjacks
Cover design by Hammond Hammond
Illustrations by Angelika Elsebach

Printed and Bound in Great Britain by Cox & Wyman Ltd.,
Reading, Berkshire

A CIP catalogue record for this book is available from
the British Library

CONTENTS

ACKNOWLEDGEMENTS

I am grateful to all those who have helped prepare this book, including my talented researchers Sarah Hamilton Fleming, Jane Ifeacho and Suzanne O'Carroll. A special word of thanks also to Anne Gains and Steven Wheeler for essential recipe testing and inspired development. I should also like to thank Liam Hamilton, Peter McHugh and Jane McCloskey at GMTV for their initial support and continuing enthusiasm. I'm also indebted to John McIlvride for producing the *Bikini Diet* television series so brilliantly. Also, thanks to Terence Renati Hairdressing for the back cover picture. Lastly, thanks to you the reader, for all your letters of inspiration. The *Bikini Diet* really works – thanks for proving it.

Liz Earle

Section 1
ON YOUR
MARKS

HOW MUCH WILL I LOSE?

This is always the very first question we ask when starting any kind of healthy eating plan. The amount of weight you will lose while following the *Bikini Diet* partly depends on how much you usually eat. The average woman consumes around 2,200 calories a day, frequently more. While following this eating plan you will be eating around 1,200 calories a day, saving at least 1,000 calories. Worked out over a single week, this amounts to around 1¹/₂lb of fat. Add to this the usual loss of water from the body during the first week of any diet and you could lose up to 7lb just after Week 1. After this, your weight-loss will be slower but just as steady. After six weeks of sticking to the eating plan you can expect to have lost up to 14lb – or a whole stone in weight!

The aim of the Bikini Diet is for you to lose a stone this summer.

MEASUREMENTS

But before beginning the *Bikini Diet*, it is important to assess realistically your current weight and find out how many pounds you should be aiming to lose. Find your current weight (in stones) and height (in feet) on the axes of the chart. Where the two points meet you will find out whether you are very overweight for your height, or if you have only a few pounds to lose.

Another more analytical way to find out if you are overweight is to calculate your own Body Mass Index or BMI. You can do this by dividing your weight by the square of your height. You'll need a calculator for this.

Start by working out your weight in kilograms (14lb in a stone; divide pounds by 2.2) and your height in metres (multiply inches by 0.025). Then divide your weight by your height and then divide again by the same figure. If you come out between 20 and 25 you are OK, but above 30 and you are clinically obese. (Any score below 20 means you are clinically underweight.)

Example: 10 stone = 140lb = 63.6 kilograms
5'4" = 64" = 1.6 metres
BMI = 24.8 – bordering on the overweight

Probably the most important measure of fatness versus thinness is your waist-to-hip ratio. Health experts now believe that fat stored above the waist is the riskiest to our future good health. Start out with the *Bikini Diet* for now, but consider a longer term weight-loss programme if your waistline is more than 80 percent of your hip measurement. A good book to follow is my *ACE Plan – Weight-loss for Life* (published by Boxtree, price £4.99). For example, if your hips measure 35", your waist should not be more than 28". This figure increases to 95 percent for men. So get out your tape measure and calculator and figure it out!

You will find your own personal *Bikini Diet* progress plan to fill in on page 22.

SO WHY DO WE GET FAT?

The obvious reason is that we eat too much and do too little. However, there is still plenty to be learned about how and why some people put on weight while others seem able to eat what they like and remain thin. Even the medical experts who specialise in treating obesity can't agree on the reasons why some of us get fat. In just a few cases, the extra weight may be to do with hormones or some other genetic factor – but these instances are very rare.

Research carried out at the Dunn Nutrition Centre in Cambridge has found that fat babies born to overweight mothers are lazier than thin ones and they move around in their cots less, so using up fewer calories. It is much more likely that overeating tends to run in families and that a person is fat because they eat too many calories and don't burn them off with exercise. Defective thyroid conditions or hormonal problems can occasionally play a part, but doctors say that this is not very common. Fatties may claim that they have a medical problem, but the reality is that they are more likely to be eating too many fattening foods.

Obesity experts, who see very overweight patients all the time, believe that our eating patterns are learned and do not come to us naturally. This means that your current relationship with food will depend a great deal on how you

YOUR WEIGHT IN STONES (1 POUND = APPROX. 0.45 KILOGRAMS)

were brought up. It can take many years for us to make behavioural changes as many overweight people have learned to override the body's hunger signals and can no longer recognise when they are hungry or full. Comfort eating is also a problem for many, which means you may eat out of a psychological need instead of a physical necessity.

Following the *Bikini Diet* is an excellent introduction to long-term, healthier eating habits. Stick with it every day for six weeks and you get the ideal incentive of seeing visible results – fast. The eating plan encourages you to count calories and fat-grams, apply portion control and get to grips with the amount of food on your plate. The inspiring recipes are nutritious as well as being extremely tasty, and use plenty of the seasonal summer fruits and vegetables that are cheap and plentiful.

THE ENERGY EQUATION

Almost all the energy that we receive from eating food is used in the body as fuel for physical activity. This includes everything from bodily functions, such as blinking the eyes, to extreme physical exercise such as running a marathon. The amount of energy that we need from our food depends almost entirely on how active we are. We measure this energy from food in terms of kilocalories (usually shortened to calories). All foods have a calorific value – the more calories it has, the more energy it can provide the body. However, if we eat lots of calories and do not burn them off as fuel for energy, the body stores the leftover calories as fat. The reason it does this is because our system may need to call up extra energy in the future and, if this happens, the body needs to have a reserve of energy it can use. All too often, however, these fat reserves simply sit around on our hips, stomachs, bottoms and thighs. So if it is all down to calories, why do some lucky people seem to be able to eat what they like and not gain any weight? Well, in reality, these fortunate few probably do not eat as much as all that. When it comes down to it, many slender folk do not have much of an interest in food. Another more important reason is down to our metabolism. Doctors and nutritionists call the amount of calories we need to get from food to keep the body ticking over our basal metabolic rate (BMR). Any other calories we eat must be used up in physical activity. Often, thin people burn up more calories to keep the body ticking over so their BMR is higher than others. Big people have a higher BMR as they have a larger body to keep going through the day.

BOOSTING THE METABOLISM

The good news is that even if we are small and do a job which doesn't use up much energy during the day, we can still increase our BMR and so boost a faster metabolism. The key to this is becoming much more physically active. This doesn't mean we all have to get to the gym every single day – it simply means using our bodies more so that we burn extra fuel. This can be on such everyday tasks as walking the dog, and taking the stairs instead of the lift. Adding extra activities, no matter how small, will burn up calories and raise your metabolism. All in all, being physically active is a very important part of any successful weight-loss plan. It doesn't always have to be taking strenuous exercise – although this can be very useful when it comes to toning and firming the body for that bikini. So, while we move on now to the most important 'food factor' part of the diet, we shall also come back to this important area with body-toning exercises on page 160.

Go for the Burn! Unless you burn up your calories you will store them as fat. Just one plain biscuit (around 70 calories) every day in excess fuel adds over 25,000 calories a year. That's more than 6lb of fat! So either burn off your biscuits by being active – or just don't eat them ...

EATING TO LOSE WEIGHT

It's important to make friends with food and not see it as the enemy. Good food builds healthy, strong, glowing bodies. It's all just a question of which foods we choose to eat! The *Bikini Diet* features tasty seasonal recipes that will help you to lose a stone this summer. However, the healthiest diet is also the one that will lead to long-term weight-loss. The *Bikini Diet* daily eating plan is both low in fats and sugars as well as high in fruits, vegetables and fibre, which is the perfect combination for increasing energy and losing excess pounds. The food pyramid chart is a good illustration of what the average weight-loss menu should look like *each day*. The guidelines for the *Bikini Diet* can be easily seen in this food pyramid, which provides an instant picture of how we should make up our meals.

Use sparingly: fats and oils. Sunflower oil contains the most vitamin E

Seldom eat: sugar, sweets and sugared drinks

Nuts and seeds are a good source of protein and are rich in vitamin E

Occasionally eat: protein such as fish, meat and poultry, milk, yoghurt and cheese

Fruits and vegetables are the best source of vitamin C and beta-carotene

Frequently eat: fruits and vegetables

Wholemeal bread is a good source of vitamin E. Baked potatoes are rich in vitamin C

Frequently eat: wholemeal bread, pasta and potatoes

* The wide bottom of the pyramid is the basis for healthy weight-loss and includes plenty of complex carbohydrates, such as wholemeal bread, brown rice and pasta.
* The next layer up on the pyramid features the fantastic variety of summer fruits and vegetables. We should also be eating plenty of these every day.

* The level above this includes the protein foods, such as fish, lean meats and chicken, eggs and cheese. We should eat a limited amount of these kinds of protein every day.
* At the top of the pyramid we find the foods that we should eat only very sparingly. These include fats and oils, try to use just a few drops of cooking oil a day, and sugary foods which we don't really need at all.

To guide you through this new way of eating, the *Bikini Diet* menus have been devised to fit in with the healthy eating food pyramid. This means that you will find plenty of wholegrains such as bread, rice and pasta, fruits, vegetables and a little protein each day. You will not find much in the way of fats and sugars as these are high in calories and will not help us to lose weight in a short space of time. Although calorie counting has its critics because it does not take into account how different types of foods are used in the body (for example, carbohydrates tend to be used as fuel, whereas fats are quickly stored), most of us are happy with the idea of counting calories. For this reason, all the recipes in the *Bikini Diet* menu plan have been calorie counted as well as analysed for their fat and fibre content, where relevant.

ALL ABOUT FATS

Of all the foods we should be most aware of, fat is the number one enemy of the trim and lean body. Fat contains the highest number of calories, at 9Kcals per gram, than any other type of food. This compares to protein (4Kcals per gram) and carbohydrate (3.75Kcals per gram). This means that it only takes a few grams of fat to start clocking up the calories. By contrast, we can eat almost *three times* as much carbohydrate – and still lose weight! This is one important reason why you will not feel hungry while following the *Bikini Diet* menu plans as they are rich in carbohydrate and low in fat.

A low-fat diet is the number one improvement you will make to achieve weight-loss for life and encourage lasting good health. Fats are the cause of excess body fat – *not* too much starch or carbohydrates. According to the Government's *Health of the Nation* report, our target for the year 2005 is to have cut our fat intake by at least 12 percent. This means that the average level of fat in the daily diet should fall from about 40 percent to no more than 35 percent. However, in order to achieve lasting weight-loss, our daily fat intake should be between 20 and 30 percent. A minimum fat intake is a fundamental part of healthy eating and is even more of a priority than the other dietary issues of sugar, fibre, salt and cholesterol intake. That is not to say that these are unimportant, just that they are secondary to the fundamental habit of eating much less fat.

The chart compares the fat content of high-fat and low-fat snacks. Remember – fat cells love fat – so don't feed it to them! In case you are worried

---

FAT CONTENT OF SNACKS

High-fat snacks

Snack	Fat per 100 grams
Brazil nuts	68g
Hazelnuts	63g
Almonds	56g
Dry roasted peanuts	49g
Cream cheese	47g
Crisps (average)	39g
Cheddar cheese	35g
Bombay mix	33g
Tortilla chips (average)	32g
Milk chocolate (average)	30g
Lower fat crisps (average)	28g
Sesame sticks	28g
Croissant	20g

Low-fat snacks

Snack	Fat per 100 grams
Plain popcorn	5.0g
Pretzels	4.5g
Plain yoghurt (average)	3.0g
Rice cakes (average)	3.0g
Bagel	1.5g
Cottage cheese (low-fat)	1.4g
Pitta bread	1.2g
Cottage cheese (very low-fat)	0.5g
Quark	0.3g
Carrots	0.3g
Banana	0.3g
Celery	0.2g
Apples	0.1g
Oranges	0.1g

---

that you will miss eating fatty foods, studies by nutrition researchers in Philadelphia found that we can all quickly teach ourselves to love a virtually fat-free diet. Over a twelve-week period, doctors found that those on a very low-fat diet reported that they actually *preferred* fat-free eating. After a period of adjustment, almost all the testers decided to continue with their new eating regime because they liked the taste of low-fat foods. So, in the long term, this way of eating is actually more enjoyable, even if it does take a few weeks to retrain the taste-buds.

FAT TYPES

All fats are made up of fatty acids and contain exactly the same number of calories. Fats and oils are equally fattening. However, some fat is far worse for building a healthy body than others. Understanding the vital differences between our everyday fats and oils makes it easy to make the changes that will lead to a leaner, healthier body. Here is the low-down on the different types of fat we eat.

Saturates

We've probably all heard that saturated fat should be avoided. The reason why a fat becomes 'saturated' has to do with its chemical composition and whether there is room on the fat molecule for hydrogen to bond on to it. Saturated fats are 'fully saturated' and have no room left for extra hydrogen to climb on board. Saturated fats are more easily recognised by being mostly solid at room temperature. Animal fats, such as butter, cheese, lard, dripping, suet and the white fat on meat (including chicken skin) are all very high in saturates. Tropical vegetable oils, such as palm kernel, palm and coconut oils are also high in saturated fats (watch out for these on the ingredient labels of biscuits, cakes and peanut butter).

Conclusion: Saturated fat is the most damaging to our health and has been clearly linked to cancer and heart disease. Cut it out of your diet.

Polyunsaturates

The polyunsaturates are literally 'very unsaturated' which means that there is plenty of room on their molecule for extra hydrogen bonds. Polyunsaturates are usually found in the form of vegetable oils. The richest sources of polyunsaturates are sunflower oil, safflower oil, corn oil and soya oil. These types of fats are thought to be less damaging to our health and they do not clog the arteries in the same way that saturated fats do. However, polyunsaturates are easily broken down by cooking and can turn into potentially dangerous peroxides, which may cause other health problems.

Recent government guidelines suggest that no more than 10 percent of our daily calories should come from polyunsaturates. This does not sound very much, but it is possible to exceed this if you use a sunflower spread on a few slices of bread a day and also use polyunsaturated oils for frying and salad dressings.

Conclusion: Small amounts of polyunsaturates are useful in the diet, but should be eaten sparingly. The more polyunsaturates you eat, the more vitamin E you need to protect the body.

Monounsaturates

The monounsaturate molecules have room for just one hydrogen atom to bond on to it. These fats are probably the healthiest of all as they do not clog the arteries in the same way that saturates can. They are also more stable during frying than the polyunsaturates, so are the best for cooking with. Monounsaturates are mostly liquid at room temperatures, but may solidify if stored in the fridge (olive oil is a good example of this). Several vegetable oils are high in monounsaturates including olive, rapeseed, groundnut (peanut), hazelnut, sesame and some blended vegetable oils.

Conclusion: Probably the best of all the fats, monounsaturates can be found in many healthy foods such as avocado, oats, nuts and seeds. One of the best all-rounders for cooking is cold-pressed olive oil, which also has a healthy amount of vitamin E.

Trans fats

These have been the subject of much of the recent research into healthy eating. Trans-fatty acids are naturally present in small amounts in meat and dairy produce. They are also artificially created by the process of hydrogenation. This is when a liquid vegetable oil is hardened by an industrial process using nitrogen and turned into a semi-solid fat. A simple example of this is when sunflower oil is hydrogenated and turned into a sunflower margarine. Unfortunately, this common procedure has the side-effect of creating a large number of trans-fatty acids. These behave in a similar way to saturated fat and have also been linked to cancer and heart disease. The trans-fatty acid content of some margarines is as high as 35 percent, but the manufacturers are not required to state this on the label. This means that those sunflower spreads that fill the chilled cabinets in supermarkets are not quite as healthy as their advertising would have us believe. Fortunately, some unhydrogenated spreads made with non-hardened oils can be found in health shops. Alternatively, choose the softest type of spread you can find, as this generally contains fewer hardened or hydrogenated oils.

Conclusion: The artificial trans-fatty acids from hydrogenated fats crop up in countless other products, including most biscuits, bread and cakes. They are best avoided, so check the label before buying any processed foods.

The recipes and menu suggestions that you will find later on do not include any hydrogenated fats and suggest the use of natural monounsaturates, such as olive oil. However, bear in mind that all vegetable oils (and most solid cooking fats and oils) are 100 percent pure fat so, no matter which you choose, they will all provide you with around 900 calories per 100g. This equals 100 calories per tablespoon.

Fat may be 'hidden' on the label in various guises. The following are all types of fat we should watch out for:

* partially hydrogenated oils
* vegetable oils
* palm oil
* shortening
* lard
* animal fat
* cream.

Slimmers should use all fats with caution and choose soft low-fat and diet spreads which are whipped with water and contain around 80 percent fat, so have slightly fewer calories. Unhydrogenated low-fat spreads are hard to find but the ultra health-conscious can track them down in good health-food shops.

COUNTING FAT-GRAMS

A healthy diet should contain no more than 35 percent fat, but a weight-loss diet should contain between 20 and 25 percent. This level will result in long-term weight-loss as well as dramatically reduce our risk of cancer and heart disease. One of the easiest ways to monitor the amount of fat we eat each day is to keep track of our fat-grams. This method of weightwatching is especially popular in America, where it has largely replaced calorie counting. There, most food labels and many restaurant menus now list their fat-gram content.

The average healthy diet consists of around 80 grams of fat a day, but this should be reduced to 20–40 grams of fat a day for dieters. Learning the fat-gram content of foods is more effective than counting calories, as it highlights the most fattening forms of foods. Read the labels and look out for fat-grams. The fat-gram content of some common foods are shown in the table, with lower-fat versions given alongside. You can work out the fat content of foods where it is not shown on the label by multiplying the number of grams of fat in a portion by nine to find out how many calories of fat a serving contains. All the recipes in the *Bikini Diet* have had their fat-grams counted for you.

ALL ABOUT CHOLESTEROL

Cholesterol is a soft, waxy substance that carries fat around the body and helps protect our vital organs. Despite the bad press cholesterol has received over the last few years, this is a vitally important substance in our bodies. The body

FAT-GRAM FINDER

Type of food	Fat-grams per portion		
Pork pie	30g		
Samosa	26g		
Streaky bacon, fried	25g	Streaky bacon, grilled	20g
Steak and kidney pie	24g		
Sausages	21g	Fat-reduced sausages	11g
Pork chop, grilled	20g		
Small beefburger	20g		
Cheddar cheese	19g	Cottage cheese	2g
Thin-cut chips	17g	Thick-cut chips	8g
Small bar of chocolate	15g		
Minced beef	14g	Minced beef, fat poured off	6g
Edam cheese	13g		
Double cream	13g	Single cream	6g
Small bag of peanuts	12g		
Roast chicken, with skin	12g	Roast chicken, without skin	4g
Fish fingers, fried	11g	Fish fingers, grilled	6g
Halva	11g		
Small bag of crisps	11g	Fat-reduced crisps	7g
Butter or margarine	8g		
Roast potatoes	8g	Boiled or baked potatoes	0g

makes its own supply in the bile ducts, so even if we cut out all cholesterol from our diet our body will continue to make the amount that it needs. Although high cholesterol levels have been linked to heart disease, the amount of dietary cholesterol we get from our foods has only a limited effect on our blood cholesterol levels. This means that many foods that contain cholesterol, such as eggs, offal and shellfish, can be safely eaten. A far more important factor is the amount of saturated fat that we eat. This type of fat does raise our blood cholesterol count and the greater the level in our blood, the more at risk we become from heart disease (the biggest cause of death in the UK).

It is estimated that about two-thirds of all adults in the UK have a blood cholesterol level that is above 5.2mmoL/L (the average target). When high cholesterol levels occur, certain oils can be useful in lowering our cholesterol score. Fish oils in the diet are important cholesterol reducers. Vegetable oils are also useful for preventing the build-up of excess cholesterol in our arteries. Some vegetable oils, such as sunflower and olive oil, are rich in the antioxidant vitamin E, which acts as a kind of detergent on the excess cholesterol and helps to prevent it from clogging the arteries. This may be one reason why Mediterranean-style diets rich in olive oil are believed to lower the risk of heart disease. So, although these oils, like all others, are high in calories, a few drops a day are very necessary for overall good health. Unlike other very low-fat diets, the *Bikini Diet* recipes include low levels of these cooking oils for good reason.

Easy ways to cut back on fat

* Switch to skimmed or semi-skimmed milk.
* Use a non-stick frying pan.
* Use a squirt of oil for frying.
* Simmer in vegetable stock instead of shallow frying in butter or lard.
* Always trim all the visible fat from meat.
* Eat more fish and poultry.
* Choose lower-fat cheeses, such as cottage cheese.
* Use low-fat yoghurt instead of evaporated milk or cream.
* Steam, grill or bake foods whenever possible instead of frying.

ALL ABOUT SUGARS

Britain is a nation of sugarholics. Confectionery sales totalling £2,332 million last year were greater than the total sum spent on bread and cereals – and the body has no need to eat any type of sugar at all! Both brown and white sugar supply only empty calories and absolutely no nourishment whatsoever. All types of sugar are also very high in calories and, after fat, are the next most powerful diet destructors. In addition to piling on the pounds, sugar is clearly linked to diseases such as diabetes. Too much refined sugar in our diet makes us more likely to put on weight and this in turn leads to a much greater risk of heart disease, strokes and high blood pressure.

As with fat, there are many different ways to describe sugar on the labels. Some believe that one type of sugar may be better for us than others, but the fact is that sugar, sucrose, glucose, dextrose and all the other 'oses' have no nutritional value other than feeding the body with empty, worthless calories. If it's energy the body needs, this is better obtained from other sources.

NOT SO SWEET NATURE

Sucrose

This is the white or brown sugar used in sweets, biscuits and cakes. Sucrose comes from sugar beet and sugar cane and is itself made up of two simpler sugars called fructose and glucose.

Fructose

This is found in sugar and honey and is the sweetest tasting sugar. Fructose tastes one-third sweeter than sucrose. Buying packets of refined fructose to use instead of refined sugar (sucrose) can save a third of our sugar calories as you will need to use less of it.

Glucose

This is naturally found in some foods and is also known as **dextrose**. Glucose gives us energy but this doesn't mean that we need sweets or sports drinks with added glucose. Our energy supplies come from complex carbohydrates, or starches, which the body breaks down into simple sugars. These are then digested and absorbed as energy. As long as we get our glucose this way we do not need to eat any type of sugar at all.

Lactose

This is the main sugar found in milk and other dairy products and is about one-third of the sweetness of sucrose.

Maltose

This sugar is manufactured from starch. As with all other sugars, the body eventually breaks it down into glucose.

None of the sugars has any place in a healthy eating or permanent weight-loss plan. Not only are all sugars high in calories, but they are also low in important nutrients. In terms of our health, the most important difference between the different types of sugars are those that are locked into the structure of a food (intrinsic sugars) and those that are added (extrinsic sugars). The intrinsic sugars can be found in the fruits and vegetables that are so plentiful in the summer. These intrinsic sugars are not harmful to our health. Extrinsic sugars are made by processing foods to release the sugars. For example, an apple contains intrinsic sugars, but turning it into processed apple purée frees the sugars and makes them extrinsic. These 'free' sugars should be used with caution. The exception is thought to be lactose which, although it is an extrinsic sugar, is not thought to damage our health. Nutritionists talk in terms of non-milk extrinsic sugars (NME) as being the types of sugars we should especially cut down on. Remember – NME is the 'enemy' and includes *all* added sugars, table sugar and concentrated fruit juices.

A 1993 report by the joint Department of Dental Public Health at London Hospital Medical College and University College London analysed the recommendations of 115 scientific studies on diet and health over the last ten years. The overwhelming majority of these advised a dramatic reduction in the amount of extrinsic sugars that we eat. Intrinsic sugars in fruits were not seen to be harmful, but the amount of extrinsic sugars (such as packet sugar, concentrated fruit juices used as food sweeteners, purées, etc.) should only amount to less than 10 percent of our total daily calories. This figure should be even lower for those wanting to achieve successful weight-loss. The good news is that naturally sweet summer fruits, such as strawberries, raspberries, melons and mangos contain only intrinsic sugars – and can be eaten as sweet, healthy treats!

It is better to snack on naturally sweet fruit instead of chocolate bars because the body deals with the two types of sugar in different ways. Eating a sugary snack which is 100 percent sugar (sucrose) means that in ten to fifteen minutes the blood sugar level will rise. This initial spurt of energy is quickly followed by a more lasting low. This is because insulin is produced when blood sugar levels are high, and this removes sugar from the bloodstream for storage in our cells. So blood sugar levels drop and leave us feeling hungrier than before. This is not a true hunger, as we only ate the sweets initially as a quick snack, but it fools the brain into believing that the stomach is empty. Sugar not only rots the teeth but can also trigger the appetite. If you have a sweet tooth and want to eat sugar, only eat it with a meal so that the rate of absorption is slowed down. Artificial sweeteners may also stimulate the appetite by triggering the release of gastric juices in the stomach in the anticipation of a raised blood glucose level. Hunger pangs may then follow as the sweeteners fail to provide any of the expected calories. For this reason it is also best to only eat chemical sweeteners at meal-times.

HOW TO STOP SUGAR CRAVINGS

* Gradually cut down the amount of sugar you use in drinks and sprinkle on cereals until you stop altogether.
* Always keep a supply of fruit nearby to snack on.
* Seedless white grapes are the sweetest fruits and will satisfy the worst sugar cravings.

* Buy reduced or no-sugar versions of foods and drinks.
* Dried fruits are high in calories because they contain concentrated fruit sugars, but a handful of raisins is still better for the body than a sugary snack.
* Carrots are also rich in natural sugars, so keep carrot sticks in the fridge for when you feel like snacking.
* When cooking, cut the amount of sugar in a recipe by at least half. You will never need as much as recipes quote. The *Bikini Diet* dessert recipes are all low in added sugar.
* Never give sugary foods or drinks to babies – they don't need them.
* Beware of ingredients ending in 'ose' such as sucrose, dextrose, etc., and of any syrups such as corn syrup.

Although the amount of packet sugar we buy has almost halved in the last decade, we are still eating more of the white stuff. This is due to the switch from home baking to convenience foods and confectionery. Most of the sugars we now eat come from processed foods and drinks, such as sweetened fruit juices and cans of fizzy drinks. When buying foods that contain sugars, always check the labels first. Ingredients must be listed in order, with the greatest first. But by dividing sugar into many different types, such as dextrose, maltose and glucose, these will appear lower down the list. When added together, you may find that sugar is actually the main ingredient. Foods labelled 'no-added sugar' or 'unsweetened' are not necessarily low in sugar. They could be foods that are naturally high in sugar or may be sweetened with concentrated fruit juices (extrinsic sugars). The table shows the amount of sugar in some products.

Food labels are often a complicated maze of weasel-words and misinformation. Check out the labels in your shopping trolley and see how many actually

SUGAR

1 level teaspoon = 5g sugar

Food	Quantity	Teaspoons
Mars bar	regular size (65g)	8.5
Coca-Cola	1 can (330ml)	7.0
Danish pastry	1 (110g)	6.5
Lucozade	small bottle (250ml)	4.5
Sugar Puffs	1 bowl (40g)	4.0
Unsweetened orange juice	1 carton (200ml)	3.5
Baked beans	1 small tin (205g)	2.5
Tinned spaghetti	1 small tin (215g)	2.0

contain sugar as the main ingredient. One of the aims of the *Bikini Diet* is to help wean you off sugar and reduce a sweet tooth and sugar cravings.

ARTIFICIAL SWEETENERS

As adding refined sugar to foods is to be avoided, are artificial sweeteners the answer? The answer has to be No. It is far better to retrain your taste-buds to accept fewer sweet foods than become dependent on a packet of chemicals.

We spend around £50 million a year on artificial sweeteners in the UK, so sugar substitutes are clearly a big business. Although they provide all the sweetness of sugar with none of the calories, there is a sour note about their safety. While most scientific studies have passed artificial sweeteners for safety, many critics believe that there is still cause for concern. Who wants to eat chemicals that the body was not designed to cope with? For example, some studies show that saccharin may increase the risk of cancer, and cyclamates have been banned from most European countries. In America, foods containing saccharin even carry a printed warning that they may be 'hazardous to your health'. The use of artificial sweeteners in processed foods has been growing at an alarming rate in recent years. Four out of five children have saccharin at least once a week, usually in the form of soft drinks and squashes. The UK allows manufacturers to add artificial sweeteners to foods and drinks together with refined sugar. This means that you or your child could be eating large amounts of these chemicals even if there is no 'diet' label on the product.

So what really goes into these handy-sized boxes of small white pills? Artificial sweeteners are essentially a cocktail of chemicals. The formula on a typical well-known brand reads like the contents of a chemistry set: sodium bicarbonate, trisodium citrate, saccharin, sodium carbonate, glycine and monosodium glutamate. No wonder they don't label the ingredients on the packet – it isn't big enough!

ALL ABOUT ALCOHOL

The final diet-breaker that must be mentioned here is alcohol. Unlike other slimming plans, the *Bikini Diet* does allow you to drink alcohol if you want to – but only in strict moderation!

Alcohol is loaded with calories so needs to be drunk with caution while following the *Bikini Diet*. Just one pint of beer contains 180 calories, so you can see how easy it is to pile on the pounds by drinking alcohol. Drinking to excess also damages your liver. This is because the liver is like a car with only one gear which always goes at the same rate. Overloading the liver with excessive drinking causes chronic damage as the liver is unable to cope with the extra quantity of alcohol. Although a small amount of 'social' drinking is unlikely to cause the liver too many problems, it will interfere with nutrient absorption. Alcohol depletes vitamin A, the B-complex vitamins, vitamin C, magnesium and zinc. In addition, drinking alcohol also encourages the body to absorb lead and aluminium. While this is not serious in the short term, you should try to eat vitamin-rich foods, such as those featured in the *Bikini Diet* Recipe section, while drinking alcohol.

YOUR BIKINI DIET ALCOHOL ALLOWANCE

While following the *Bikini Diet* menu plan you are allowed to drink three small glasses of wine (or their equivalent) each week. It is best to spread this throughout the week and not drink your allowance in one evening. Once you have completed the menu plan, you should limit your alcohol intake to sensible levels in order to maintain your weight-loss. The Health Education Authority advises that women should drink no more than twenty-one units and men no

ALCOHOL - CALORIES AND UNITS

Beer, lager and cider	Calories	Units of Alcohol
Half pint (284ml, 10floz) of:		
Bitter	90	1
Brown ale	80	1
Strong ale or lager	85	2
Low-alcohol lager	60	0.25
Dry cider	95	1
Sweet cider	110	1
Strong cider	100	2
Wine		
Average small glass (113ml, 4floz) of:		
Dry white wine	75	1
Rosé	85	1
Sweet white wine	85	1
Champagne	70	1
Fortified Wine		
1 pub measure (50ml, 1/3 gill) of:		
Dry sherry or similar	55	1
Medium sherry	60	1
Cream sherry	70	1
Spirits		
1 single measure (25ml, 1/6 gill) of:		
brandy, whisky, gin, rum or vodka	50	1

more than twenty-eight units, spread throughout a week (see table). Women have a lower allowance than men because of the differing water content in their bodies. In men, between 55 and 65 percent of the body weight is made up of water. In women, this figure is between 45 and 55 percent. Alcohol is distributed throughout the body fluids, so in men it is more 'diluted' than in women. In addition, a woman's liver is smaller and more likely to suffer damage.

WHAT'S IN A DRINK?

Keep a track on what you drink with the table (see left). If you're concerned about your drinking, switch to low-alcohol lagers, drink de-alcoholised wine or make spritzers with white wine and sparkling mineral water. Low-calorie mixers such as tonic and bitter lemon are also good options.

Another problem with drinking alcohol is that it reduces the amount of water within the system. This is because alcohol blocks the action of an antidiuretic hormone, so the more you drink, the more dehydrated you become. The way to drink healthily is to drink slowly, and to match each alcoholic drink with a large glass of water. This ensures that fluid is put back into the system to replace the water lost by drinking alcohol. Water is especially important for good health and weight-loss. Often overlooked, it is important not to forget to drink plenty of water on a daily basis. Water is a natural detoxifier, helping to sluice out the build-up of toxins inside the system by binding them with the fibre from our summer fruits and vegetables.

Drinking water half an hour before a meal also gives you a temporary sense of fullness and helps prevent hunger pangs. The best time to drink water is half an hour before or after a meal. This allows time for food to be efficiently digested by the concentrated acids in the stomach. Try to drink water throughout the day instead of one or two very large glassfuls in one go.

Remember – if you feel thirsty, your body probably dehydrated twenty minutes ago. Tap water contains nitrates, chlorine, aluminium and other substances, so it is worth investing in a filter jug, and never use water from the hot tap as it is constantly reheated which affects its mineral content. It helps to keep a large bottle of low-sodium (salt) mineral water on your desk or in the kitchen and aim to finish it every day.

AND FINALLY ...

Now we know all we need to about the foods and drinks to be watched or avoided, such as fats, sugars and alcohol, it's time to look to the foods that will ensure our success in losing the pounds this summer. The good news is that there are plenty of foods that help us to lose weight quickly, safely and easily. Just continue to the next section to find out how these super-foods will help YOU!

Section 2
GET SET...

Now you are ready to begin the *Bikini Diet*. But, before starting, let's get ready for weight-loss. The first step is to keep a record of your present weight and vital statistics, so you can monitor your progress over the coming weeks.

YOUR PERSONAL BIKINI DIET PROGRESS PLAN

Date started: ..../........../..........

Weight on starting: ....stone ....lb (.........kg)

Statistics on starting: bust ....in (.........cm)

waist ....in (.........cm)

hips ....in (.........cm)

Weight at end of Week 1: ....stone ....lb (.........kg)

Weight at end of Week 2: ....stone ....lb (.........kg)

Weight at end of Week 3: ....stone ....lb (.........kg)

Weight at end of Week 4: ....stone ....lb (.........kg)

Weight at end of Week 5: ....stone ....lb (.........kg)

Weight at end of Week 6: ....stone ....lb (.........kg)

Statistics at end of Week 6: bust ....in (.........cm)

waist ....in (.........cm)

hips ....in (.........cm)

Total weight lost: ....stone ....lb (.........kg)

Total inch loss: ....in (.........cm)

BIKINI DIET SUPER-FOODS

In the previous section we looked at all the diet breakers, such as fats, sugars and alcohol. Now let's take a look at the many diet makers. These are the super-foods that help to boost our vitality and energy levels whilst also helping to shift the pounds. You can see from the *Bikini Diet* food pyramid on page 9 that eating plenty of carbohydrates is the basis for your new weight-loss regime. Carbohydrates are 'super-foods' because the body stores any extra carbohydrate we eat in the form of glycogen. The body cannot make much glycogen from fatty foods. This means that the body resists making extra fat from carbohydrates until its glycogen stores are replenished. It is very hard for the body to turn carbohydrates into fat.

All nutritionists agree that one of the most important rules of any weight-loss or healthy eating plan is to eat *much* more in the way of carbohydrates because they are packed with fibre. One of the many reasons why the *Bikini Diet* menus work is because they focus on high-fibre carbohydrates that make us to feel full on fewer calories. High-fibre foods also tend to be low in fat and sugar – another good reason why they are the perfect partner for successful slimming. The bottom line is that we all need fibre. Too little fibre in our daily diet results in the bowels becoming sluggish and constipated. This then leads to further problems such as varicose veins, gallstones and piles. In the longer term, a low-fibre diet increases the risk of colon cancer as the body is unable to eliminate toxins effectively and speedily.

Fibre Providers

Unfortunately, the average diet has dramatically changed during the last decade. We are eating far more processed foods such as white bread, refined fats and sugars than ever before. We have given up our previous dietary staples, including oats, barley and lentils in favour of low-fibre, convenience foods. By contrast, those living in Mediterranean countries, such as the Spanish and the Italians, have continued to eat the same foods for thousands of years. The southern Europeans eat many more fresh fruits, vegetables and whole grains in the form of breads and pasta. This has meant a much lower incidence of chronic disease, such as heart disease and cancer. Fibre provides the broom to give our insides a thorough sweep and cleans out the colon where some of the most dangerous diseases breed. Eating more fibre is important, not only for effective weight-loss but also for better health, increased vitality and energy levels.

Adding fibre-rich foods to our everyday meals is simple, inexpensive and very easy. Wholegrain cereals provide about ten times as much fibre as ordinary corn-flakes, so a simple switch in your breakfast bowl can dramatically boost your fibre intake. Adding a handful of freshly chopped vegetables to soups or eating potatoes with their skins on also makes the most of the natural fibre in cheap, plentiful foods. Eating refined grains such as white flour, however, does not work so well because this has had the outer husk stripped away during food processing. Not only does this remove our fibre, it also leaches away many of the valuable vitamins found in the fibrous husk or 'germ' of wheat. This is why many of the *Bikini Diet* recipes include wholemeal bread, brown rice and wholewheat pasta.

FIBRE FACTS

Wholemeal bread and whole grains are probably the first things we think of as being high in fibre. But summer's vitamin-rich fruits and vegetables are also some of our very best sources. Fibre is basically a carbohydrate that is broken down in the intestine and it comes in several different guises. It consists of the cellulose fibres that form the structure of green, leafy vegetables and the outer skins of sweetcorn and beans. There are two types of fibre: *soluble* fibre, which is soft and spongy and *insoluble* fibre, which is coarse and hard.

Soluble fibre is essential for successful weight-loss as it dissolves in the liquids in the stomach and helps to fill us up and prevent hunger pangs. Soluble fibre is also important in the upper portion of the gut where it slows down the absorption of nutrients from food. This is no bad thing, as it allows time for vital vitamins and nutrients to work their way into the bloodstream before the food passes into the colon. Soluble fibre is also vital for regulating the release of glucose into the bloodstream. This means we avoid hunger pangs and sudden sugar cravings as our blood sugars are stabilised. The best way to avoid an attack of the munchies is to make sure we eat plenty of soluble fibre from fruits, vegetables and oats.

STOCKING UP

Before you get going with the *Bikini Diet* menu plan, make sure you have all the ingredients handy. If you can, buy a few weeks' supply before you start. This way you'll be spending less time in the supermarket shopping for foods which may tempt you into buying fattening goodies which aren't on your *Bikini Diet* shopping list.

YOUR BIKINI DIET SHOPPING LIST
Carbohydrates

These group of foods are an important part of successful slimming, so make sure you have plenty of supplies in the store-cupboard. It's easy to stock up with these foods, so you always have a good selection to choose from.

Rice – not just plain white rice, try buying several varieties and cooking them together for a change. The Italian arborio risotto rice makes deliciously creamy savoury dishes. Wild rice is also good to combine with other varieties, although it takes longer to cook. Try the new red rices from the

BREAKFAST CEREAL CHART

(measurements in grams per 100g)

Cereal	Total Fats	Total Sugars	Kcal
All Bran	2.5	19	261
Bran Flakes	1.6	18.7	318
Coco Pops	0.9	38.2	384
Oat Bran Flakes	2.4	16.8	357
Corn Flakes	0.5	8.2	360
Crunchy Nut Corn Flakes	3.8	36.3	398
Frosties	0.4	41.9	377
Muesli (average)	5.2	26.2	363
Muesli (no added sugar)	7.4	15.7	366
Porridge (made with water)	1.0	Almost Nil	49
Porridge (made with full-fat milk)	4.7	4.7	116
Puffed Wheat	1.0	0.3	321
Ready Brek (plain)	6.6	1.7	373
Rice Krispies	0.8	10.6	369
Ricicles	0.5	41.9	381
Shredded Wheat	2.2	0.8	325
Shreddies	1.1	10.2	331
Smacks	1.5	50.0	386
Special K	0.9	17.2	377
Start	1.4	29.1	355
Sugar Puffs	0.6	56.5	324
Weetabix	2.0	5.2	352
Weetos	1.9	33.2	372

Camargue in southern France. These are nutty, aromatic and a rich ruby shade. Brown rices come in several shapes and forms from health-food shops. Nutty and filling, the organic varieties are often tastier than the brands usually found in supermarkets. Try organic long-grain, short-grain and brown Basmati rices cooked together. Health-food shops also sell Whole Earth precooked tinned brown rice, which tastes good and is a great time-saver.

Potatoes – no, these are not fattening! It all depends on how you cook them. Plain boiled potatoes are low in calories and high in vitamin C. They also provide plenty of fibre if you keep the skins on. Jacket potatoes are a quick and tasty standby, and the *Bikini Diet* includes several instant, low-calorie fillings. The best way to prepare jacket potatoes is to microwave them until almost cooked, then crisp the skins in a hot oven for ten to fifteen minutes. Choose organically grown potatoes when possible as these are grown in mineral-rich soil and are not sprayed with antisprouting chemicals.

Bread – the best breads to buy are wholemeal as these are made with the 'whole' germ of the wheat grain. Several organically grown brands are available and these tend to have a lower pesticide content as their wheat is not sprayed with chemicals before processing. Wholemeal breads are high in fibre and are more filling than white breads, so it's worth switching to wholemeal while you are on a weight-loss regime.

Pasta – as with bread, it's worth choosing wholemeal pasta to fill you up more quickly. There are so many shapes and sizes to choose from – you can now cook pasta every night without getting bored! Pasta itself is low in calories (the problem is usually with the sauces and cheese toppings), and the *Bikini Diet* features several tasty low-calorie pasta dishes. It's also fun to experiment with more unusual ingredients, such as buckwheat pasta (from health-food shops) and rice noodles.

Breakfast cereals – these are a quick and easy way to start the day, so are included in the *Bikini Diet* daily menu plans. All boxes of cereal have an information panel printed on the side, and it's worth reading this before buying as some contain masses of sugar. Your daily menu plans include Weetabix, Puffed Wheat and puffed rice cereals as these have very little added salt and sugar. For a more comprehensive comparison, see the breakfast cereal ingredient table on the previous page.

Low-fat foods

Milk – dairy products such as milk and cheese are good for the body as they are rich in bone-building calcium. This is important for women to ward off bone-thinning osteoporosis. However, they can also be very high in fat so choose carefully. Full-fat milk contains 22g of fat per pint, semi-skimmed has 11g per pint and skimmed milk contains just 1g of fat. It is well worth switching to semi-skimmed milk instead of full fat and, once your taste-buds have adapted, try skimmed milk on cereal and in tea or coffee.

Cheese – all cheese is high in fat – even the 'lower fat' versions! If you want to lose weight, you will have to cut down on your fat intake, and this includes cheese. Cottage cheese, especially the low-fat varieties, is a good substitute and can be spread on crackers and crispbreads for an instant snack. Add a handful of chopped herbs and a clove of crushed garlic to make a delicious instant dip.

Spreads – use low-fat spreads on bread or toast, checking the labels before you buy to see which brands contain the least number of fat-grams. Low-fat spreads are whipped with water and so contain fewer of the high calorie oils. If you look in health-food shops you can even find unhydrogenated low-fat spreads (see page 13), which are probably the healthiest choice.

Yoghurt – low-fat yoghurt and fromage frais are also good choices and excellent substitutes in recipes using cream, sour cream or cream cheese. The *Bikini Diet* menu plan includes delicious summer dessert ideas using very low-fat fromage frais and yoghurts which contain only a fraction of the fat of normal puddings, without sacrificing any of the taste! Check the table to see how you can easily cut back on fat.

FAT FACTS

Cream		Fromage Frais		Yoghurt	
Double	50% fat	Plain	7% fat	Greek	7% fat
Whipping	40%	Fruit	6%	Natural	1.5%
Single	19%	Very low-fat	0.5%	Low-fat	0.8%

Summer produce

Salad – the most popular slimming summer meal must be the salad. These days there are so many different varieties of lettuces, tomatoes and other salad ingredients available that we are spoilt for choice. Save preparation time by washing and sorting lettuce leaves in bulk. Mix together different varieties such as bitter batavia, frisée and endive with crispy sweet iceberg or little gem and store in plastic bags in the fridge ready for instant use. This works out much cheaper than buying prepacked salads and is very convenient.

Vegetables – most vegetables are cheap and plentiful during the summer months, so there is no excuse for not treating the family to a wide variety. Vegetables such as carrots, celery, fennel, cucumber and pea pods are delicious raw, so keep a plastic box full of an assortment in the fridge for when you feel like nibbling.

Fruits – summer's fruits are also in abundance, so make the most of the current glut of strawberries, raspberries and other soft fruits. Tropical fruits are also cheaper at this time of year, so explore the taste sensations of mango, papaya, kiwi, lychees, kumquat, persimmon and pomegranate. You will find recipes using unusual fruits in the *Bikini Diet* Recipe section.

Snacks and extras

Inevitably, one of the hardest parts about being on a diet is the feeling that you can't afford to snack between meals. Rigid discipline is hard to stick to, especially when we need to satisfy hunger pangs. The *Bikini Diet* recognises this fact of life and makes some allowance for snacking. In addition to your fridgeful of salad bits and carrot sticks, make sure you also have other low-calorie and low-fat treats in stock. Rice cakes are a great low-fat snack and are good to crunch on instead of a biscuit that is high in fat and loaded with sugar. You can find many different varieties and flavours, such as sesame and corn, in all good health-food shops. Sauces and dressings are also useful ways to boost the flavour of otherwise bland foods, such as baked potatoes and plain rice. I use a teaspoon of bottled garlic sauce to enliven baked potato skins and stir a splash of passata (sieved tomatoes) into rice and pasta dishes. Watch out for high-calorie mayonnaise and salad cream. Switch to low-fat versions or, better still, buy some balsamic or cider vinegar and use small amounts of this to flavour salads with instead. Freshly squeezed lemon juice is also a good way to add flavour to many foods without adding any calories.

SUPPLEMENTARY BENEFITS

Unfortunately there are no short cuts to losing weight. The only way to slim successfully is to get used to eating plenty of the *Bikini Diet* foods, instead of the high-fat, sugary foods most of us tend to live on. It is also important to eat less, and to keep on eating less for a considerable time (which is why all the *Bikini Diet* recipes are carefully counted and measured). Anyone who tries to tell you otherwise is more interested in relieving you of the pounds in your purse than the pounds on your thighs!

There's an endless array of products and programmes on the market which claim to have special powers to help you lose weight. Look in the tabloid Sunday papers and you'll often see full-page advertisements for products that promise super-fast, effortless weight-loss. In the classified sections of some magazines you'll find ads for clinics specialising in doctor-supervised weight-loss programmes using various medications. You may even be approached directly by salespeople promoting diet pills. Beware! They don't always deliver what they promise.

SLIMMING SCAMS

Sadly, with so many people desperate to lose weight there are easy fortunes to be made by the unscrupulous. An advertisement that dangles the carrot of fast weight-loss without the discipline of a calorie-controlled diet will bring the cheques pouring in. Trading Standards Officers are all too familiar with complaints about mail-order products that claim to aid slimming but which turn out to be ineffective. So don't get caught by the con artists.

One of the biggest slimming scams the UK has ever seen ended in 1994, when the family who marketed Bai Lin tea were finally brought to justice after grossing what has been estimated to be millions of pounds selling yellow boxes of Chinese tea – that experts declared had no weight-reducing qualities whatsoever. Bai Lin tea was widely promoted by advertisements in the national press, featuring such claims as:

Bye bye fat. Buy Bai Lin. No more dieting. Eat normal meals.

Just drinking the tea three times a day after normal meals can rip off the kilos.

After literally thousands of complaints, it still took nearly eight years to secure a prosecution under the Trade Descriptions Act, during which time nearly a million hapless dieters had parted with £4.95 per pack.

HOW TO GET VALUE FOR MONEY

If you bear in mind the following information, you should be more likely to get your money's worth.

1. Whatever anyone says – it's only possible to lose weight by eating fewer calories than you use up. Unless you undertake a long-term programme of very regular, vigorous exercise you're unlikely to noticeably boost your body's energy demands. So, for most people, losing weight means eating less over a sustained period of time. If an advertisement, label or salesperson says that their particular product will let you eat what you like and still lose weight, be suspicious. If, on the other hand, the small print tells you that this product can only work as part of a calorie-controlled diet, then you should ask yourself whether you might not be better off just following a calorie-controlled diet anyway – without buying the product.

2. Products that guarantee you will lose weight from particular areas of the body ('spot reduction'), should likewise be treated with caution. Everyone is different, and so loses weight at different rates from various parts of the body. No responsible manufacturer would mislead consumers with promises they cannot fulfil.

3. 'Stay slim for good' is another promise that cannot be guaranteed. Permanent weight-loss is possible, but it depends upon the successful slimmer changing his or her eating habits for good, because if you go back to your old eating habits then before long you'll be re-united with your old figure.

4. Specific medical claims, for example, 'speeds fat burning', 'boosts metabolism', 'appetite suppressant' or offering relief from medical conditions (such as diabetes or high blood pressure) may be breaking the law. If in doubt, check with your local Trading Standards Officer.

The following section is a useful guide through the maze of the most commonly promoted types of pills and potions, and you should get a better understanding how they are supposed to work, and why, in some cases, they may not.

MEDICAL PRODUCTS

There are certain medications, available on prescription only, which are occasionally used to aid weight-loss. The pharmaceutical approach to tackling obesity is to use one of two tactics:

* Reduce hunger, so you don't feel inclined to eat so much and thus find it easier to stick to a diet.
* Increase energy expenditure, so that you can lose weight without altering your current diet.

Reduce hunger

Doctors occasionally prescribe amphetamines as an aid to weight-loss. These drugs work by stimulating the central nervous system and suppressing appetite. Familiar brand names in this category are Tenuate dospan, Duromine, Ionamin and Apisate. Amphetamines are addictive, so should be reserved for cases of severe obesity and used only for short periods in conjunction with a calorie-controlled diet, as a means of starting the patient off on their weight-loss programme. Amphetamines can produce a range of side-effects that may include sleeplessness, nervousness, dry mouth, headaches, agitation, high blood pressure and even psychotic states and hallucinations. If used for prolonged periods tolerance develops – the drug needs to be taken in greater and greater quantities to produce the same effect.

Any doctor who hands out amphetamines for weight-loss in anything other than severe, health-threatening obesity and who repeats prescriptions over prolonged periods could be acting unethically.

There have been numerous reports of doctors operating private weight-loss clinics in which drugs such as those named above are dispensed more or less on demand, in exchange for a fee. One national newspaper carried an exposé, after despatching a team of undercover reporters – all young, healthy, underweight women – to a number of clinics. They were sold these potentially dangerous drugs with little or no medical checks. Alarmingly, the day after the report appeared in the paper the editorial offices were inundated with calls from overweight readers desperate to contact the clinics so that they, too, could buy the drugs.

The most widely used prescription drug in the treatment of obesity is dexfenfluramine (brand name Adifax). This works by making the food you eat more satisfying, so you end up eating less. Though safer than amphetamines, dexfenfluramine does not guarantee weight-loss, and it often only produces results in the short term – weight-loss often grinds to a halt after a number of months; and, as with any diet, if the dieter goes back to overeating after discontinuing treatment then the weight will be regained. This treatment should be reserved for people with difficult weight problems that have not responded to conventional diets, and used as a 'kick start' to a longer-term, calorie-controlled diet programme.

Increase energy expenditure

Drug companies continue to search for the elusive ingredient that will speed up metabolic rates so that people can lose weight without changing their normal eating habits. There's every reason to believe that one day they'll succeed, but the state of current research suggests that we are still many years away from a breakthrough.

NON-MEDICAL SLIMMING PILLS, PATCHES AND POTIONS

Proprietary slimming aids range from medically proven products, such as vitamin and mineral supplements, to ineffective and even dangerous gimmicks.

It is against the law for a product or programme to make claims suggesting it's possible to lose weight except by taking in fewer calories than your body needs. The only other claims that are allowed with regard to weight-loss are either for diuretics (products that make you shed excess water creating a temporary illusion of weight-loss) or for slimmer's vitamin and mineral supplements, inasmuch as these can help you get the nutrition you need while you are eating less. Any other promises are likely to be insupportable ... and illegal. Slimming aids you can buy or might see advertised include the following types:

* meal replacements and very low-calorie diets
* fibre or bulking agents
* herbal products
* slimming patches
* gums, fat blockers and starch blockers
* fat-burners and metabolic enhancers.

Formula meal replacements and very low-calorie diets (VLCDs)

These are designed to replace a specified number of meals per day (in the case of VLCDs, to replace all your meals) with calorie-counted, nutritionally fortified formula drinks or snacks. If you find it difficult or inconvenient to prepare nutritionally balanced low-calorie meals day in, day out, then you may find these helpful because the meals are quick to make up and the calories and nutrition are worked out for you. However, they do not help you to retrain your eating habits, or get you used to the idea of shopping for, cooking and preparing healthy, low-calorie meals. Formulas that claim to include 'fat burners' or ingredients that speed up metabolism should be treated with suspicion.

Fibre tablets or bulking agents

These include chewable tablets or pastilles that are taken before a meal with a glass of water. The bulking ingredient is supposed to suck in water like a sponge, swelling in the stomach and so giving a feeling of fullness. The result should be that you are inclined to eat less food at your meal. There are also high-fibre drinks which produce the same effect and which can be taken as a snack between meals.

Some people do find this type of product helps them stick to their diet, but the effectiveness of bulking agents depends on why and how you overeat. For example, if your weight problem is caused by nibbling between meals, then a bulking agent taken at meal times only is unlikely to tackle the root cause of the problem.

Some herbal tablets include glucomannan fibre, which absorbs more than ten times as much water as wheat bran and so is a highly effective bulking agent. Programmes including glucomannan have been shown to result in weight-losses without any apparent change in eating habits (of course, the weight-loss only results because the slimmer is actually eating less food thanks to the feeling of fullness – the value of the product is that it can produce this result without making you conscious of deprivation).

On the same principle, wheat bran was until quite recently widely recommended for its natural bulking action. In fact, large quantities of bran, which is indigestible, can absorb minerals as it passes through the digestive tract and can, in extreme cases, lead to mineral deficiencies. Some doctors talk of the so-called 'muesli belt syndrome', reputedly caused by eager parents feeding their children so much high-fibre breakfast cereal that they became malnourished. So avoid sprinkling raw bran on to everything. Healthier natural dietary bulk is produced by the fibre in vegetables, oats, lentils and beans.

Herbal remedies

Herbal preparations, such as boldo, generally act as mild diuretics or water tablets. That is, they encourage the body to eliminate excess body fluids. This is not an effective strategy for long-term weight-loss!

A diuretic, whether included in a herbal remedy or medically prescribed, may well make you appear to shed several pounds in a couple of days. The trouble is, it is just water, not fat. So it is just a short-term effect. You can only carry a limited amount of excess fluid, and once that has been flushed out the weight-loss will stop. You won't have lost any fat and before long the excess fluid will creep straight back on again.

If you tend to retain water before a period, and this time coincides with the night you are due to wear your slinkiest little black dress, then herbal products that use euphemisms like 'cleanse the system', 'eliminate excess body fluids' and 'flush out toxins' could make the dress a slightly more comfortable fit on the night. But such products have no effect on your body fat. The only way to get rid of that is to eat less.

Slimming patches

So-called 'slimming patches' are similar in appearance to the nicotine patches that are often successful in helping smokers. The slimming variety, which often contain seaweed extracts, are supposed to slow-release compounds into the skin which then aid weight-loss. There is no clinical evidence whatsoever to support these claims. In fact, a leading expert in herbal and homoeopathic medicines was recently quoted as saying that slimming patches 'misuse the concept of homoeopathic medicine in the most irresponsible way'. Patch users are advised to follow a calorie-controlled diet at the same time, as any weight-loss can only result from this.

Gums, 'fat blockers' and 'starch blockers'

Steer well clear of any product that claims to prevent absorption of some or all of the food you eat by lining the digestive tract. These have been sold under an ever-changing variety of brand names by mail order through advertisements in the tabloid press.

Such products are generally based on a natural ingredient called guar gum which, when taken before a meal, forms a viscous gel that delays stomach emptying and slows the absorption of carbohydrate from the intestine. Although it may occasionally be prescribed by doctors in specific clinical situations (e.g. diarrhoea, diabetes) it is not safe for general use and is more likely to produce unpleasant gastrointestinal effects, the least of which are wind and abdominal bloating, than weight-loss.

Fat-burners and metabolic enhancers

A number of products claim to enhance fat burning or to quicken metabolic rate – and therefore enable you to lose weight without making significant changes to your eating habits.

Be assured that, to date, there is no clinical evidence that any product or ingredient is capable of achieving this effect reliably and safely in humans. Furthermore, if the claims were true, the product would by law need to have a medical licence and be supplied under strict medical supervision only. So when you see off-the-page advertisements for products making outlandish claims, just turn the page and save your money.

Fat Magnets

These new slimming supplements are designed to bind with some of the fats in the food we consume, and convert it to a form of fat that passes harmlessly through the digestive system without being absorbed. The active ingredient in Fat Magnets is ChitosanPlex which is a version of chitosan, a substance made from the powdered shells of shrimps, crabs and other crustacea. ChitosanPlex is an amino polysaccharide which literally has a magnetic effect on certain fats. Ingested fat has a negative charge which is attracted to the positive charge of ChitosanPlex. Each 500mg has been shown in trials to absorb over 4 times its own weight in fat, but it is unable to distinguish between 'good' and 'bad' types of fat. As we have seen, we all need a certain amount of essential fatty acids in the diet. For this reason, dieters are recommended to aim to trap only a percentage of the fats they consume – between 30 percent and 50 percent. Of course, Fat Magnets are no replacement for a healthy well-balanced diet, but they may be able to aid those who find it difficult to cut down their fat intake. See Useful Addresses for details. Other supplements containing chitosan and chitin are also increasingly available.

AromaTrim™

The therapeutic effects of essential oils are well documented and this new product from America is designed to aid weight-loss by controlling food cravings and suppressing appetite between meals. The pack contains two different blends of essential oils; *Suppress* is made up of fennel, hickory, aniseed and mint, and *Crave Ender* which contains fennel and grapefruit. The Suppress cartridge should be inhaled whenever you feel the urge to snack while the Crave Ender should only be used with food. If you are desperate for some chocolate, pizza, fries or any fattening foods not allowed on the *Bikini Diet*, inhale the aroma as you begin to tuck into the diet breaker. Then continue to inhale until the taste of the food begins to change and you no longer have the desire to eat. For further details see Useful Addresses on page 180.

NEWCOMERS

Research is continuing into ingredients that might be able to enhance weight-loss. A number of products currently sold through health-food outlets attempt to do this, based on various principles. None to date have been proven as successful but are the subject of continuing research and may well eventually be deemed to have some benefit to dieters. Many are expensive though, so do not part with your money unless you are prepared to be disappointed.

A great deal of interest has been generated in the last couple of years by HCA, or alpha-hydroxycitrate, a natural ingredient extracted from the tamarind fruit. HCA has been found in a number of published experiments to suppress hunger and reduce the rate of fat synthesis ... in rats. To date, though, there is no reliable evidence that the results can be replicated in humans.

My Slimming Supplement chart lists other potential diet-product ingredients.

SLIMMING SUPPLEMENT CHART

Ingredient	Comment
Acetyl-L-Carnitine	An amino acid, used in fat metabolism – it transports fatty acids to the mitochondria (the cell's 'furnaces') where they are burnt for energy. In laboratory tests on isolated muscle tissue, it seems to help muscle performance. No clinical evidence that supplements are of benefit in weight-loss.
Chromium	Used in the metabolism of sugar, can help with control of blood sugar levels in diabetes. May have a role in controlling appetite.
Co-enzyme Q10	In clinical tests improves the capacity for physical work, and is an effective antioxidant nutrient. No clinical evidence that supplements are of benefit in weight-loss.
Dahlulin (extract of dahlia)	A type of fibre, believed to slow down energy release from complex carbohydrates, smoothing peaks and troughs in blood sugar levels. When taken in sufficient quantities with other food may reduce likelihood of rebound fatigue or carbohydrate cravings.
Enzyme preparations	When taken in a nutritional supplement, may help make other nutrients more bioavailable if included in sufficient quantities. No clinical evidence that supplements are of benefit in weight-loss.
Fructose	Fructose (fruit sugar) is a simple sugar that is used by the body in a slightly different way to the sugars usually found in sweet snacks (glucose) or ordinary sugar (sucrose). It produces smaller peaks and troughs in blood sugar levels, so if taken in place of other sugars it may be less likely to stimulate rebound fatigue or carbohydrate cravings.
Ginkgo biloba	Can increase blood flow, enhancing the supply of oxygen to the tissues. May have antioxidant nutrient properties but no clinical evidence that supplements are of benefit in weight-loss.
L-ornithine	An amino acid. Believed to stimulate muscle growth in preference to fat production. No clinical evidence that supplements are of benefit in weight-loss.

TRIED AND TESTED

Instead of wasting your money on unproven products with spurious claims, stick with the *Bikini Diet* and watch the pounds drop off. Each daily menu is calorie counted to provide up to 1,200 calories a day. This is a sensible calorie restriction which will get results fast without leaving you feeling tired, hungry or undernourished. All the recipes are based around high-vitality foods that have large amounts of energy-giving vitamins, minerals, enzymes and other essential nutrients. All the recipes are also quick and easy to prepare – who wants to spend the summer in the kitchen?

The recipes are nutritious, delicious and very filling – so no need to endure the hunger pangs of so many other diets. Because these recipes include lots of carbohydrates they will quickly make you feel full. You will be enjoying plenty of starchy foods such as bread, potatoes, pasta and rice, as well as seasonally cheap fruits and vegetables. As with all well-planned diets, this eating plan is very low in fat and sugar, which will help you adjust your long-term eating habits to make sure that your summer weight-loss stays off all year round.

Section 3

GET SET TO FOOD COMBINE

Food combining is an eating plan designed to allow us to get the best from our food by not mixing 'the foods that fight'. It is widely used by supermodels (including Claudia Schiffer) as a way of giving weight-loss an extra boost. Food combining encourages us to eat as many fresh fruit and vegetables as possible and to never mix starch with protein as this is thought to interfere with our digestive processes. The concept of food combining for health originated in America in the nineteenth century from Dr Howard Hay. This pioneering doctor was way before his time in believing what we now know to be true, 'that the body is merely a composite of what goes into it daily in the form of food and drink'. It is this belief that prompted him to develop the system of eating which made him famous – the Hay system of food combining. Dr Hay thought that all diseases are caused by the wrong chemical conditions in the body. He said that eating the wrong mixture of foods leads to an over-accumulation of acids (the natural end-products of digestion and metabolism) and that this is responsible for the wrong chemical conditions. As the body is unable to eliminate these acids they decay inside the body, harming it.

To avoid this build-up of toxic acids within the body, Dr Hay advised his patients to avoid eating much meat and too many refined carbohydrates (e.g. sugar and products made from white flour). According to his theory, we build up a tolerance to eating these 'bad' foods and this reduces our vitality. He found that after adopting his system of eating, those that return to their previous eating habits your stomach will immediately react to the 'bad' food.

He had a theory for weight-loss too and maintained that storing toxins internally can cause weight-gain. A build-up of toxins, such as pesticides and pollution, can occur in the body which is usually stored in our fat cells well away from the vital organs. It is these toxins stored near the surface of the skin which may be partly responsible for the orange-peel skin we know as cellulite. In addition, these toxins are acidic, so our bodies retain water to neutralise the acid, giving us a bloated appearance. This build-up of trapped toxins has an accumulative effect on the body and if we continue to hamper our digestive system by eating junk food and, according to Dr Hay, combining the foods that fight, the store of toxic waste can continue to grow, making it difficult to lose weight.

One of the great benefits of food combining is that you can eat as much of the right foods as you want and still lose weight! The food combining recipes contain a wide range of fruits and vegetables which have a high water content. The human body is made of a staggering 70 percent water and to maintain a healthy body, we need to continually replenish our supplies of water. It makes sense, therefore, to eat foods which are high in water. Other foods are concentrated, meaning that the water content has been removed, either through processing or through cooking. The most healthy and effective way of losing weight is by adopting a diet that is 70 percent fruits and vegetables and only 30 percent concentrated foods such as grains, meat, fish and legumes (pulses).

HOW FOOD COMBINING WORKS

The most important rule to remember when food combining is not to mix carbohydrates with proteins or fruit acids. **Proteins** refer to concentrated animal proteins such as meat, poultry, fish and cheese. **Carbohydrates** are concentrated starches, such as grains, bread, cereals and potatoes. Sugars also fall into this category. Following this fundamental principle of food combining, here are five basic rules of thumb:

* Starches and sugars should not be eaten with proteins at the same meal
* The diet should consist mainly of vegetables, salads and fruits
* All processed and refined foods should be avoided and ideally only wholegrain carbohydrates should be eaten, such as wholemeal bread, pasta and brown rice. White flour, sugar and processed fats, in particular, should be avoided
* Proteins, starches and animal fats should be eaten in moderation only
* There should be at least a four-hour interval between a starch and protein meal.

STARCH AND PROTEIN DIGESTION

Dr Hay had good reason for advising his patients not to combine starch and protein in the same meal. He maintained that when animal proteins reach the stomach, the body releases hydrochloric acid, which activates the enzyme known as pepsin. This enzyme has the important job of splitting and absorbing the proteins and the process can only take place in a completely acid environment. Eating carbohydrates upsets the acid medium and this interferes with the digestion of proteins. Followers of the Hay system believe the undigested protein can have a serious impact on our health and our ability to lose weight, because the body is unable to utilise it and may have trouble removing the leftover waste effectively.

Similarly, the body is thought to require an alkaline medium in order to digest carbohydrates. Digestion is initiated in the mouth by the action of the enzyme ptyalin, which splits the starches before they enter the small intestine where they are digested further. (It is important that all foods are thoroughly chewed otherwise the small intestine will be unable to digest food properly.) In the stomach, saliva containing the active ptyalin is mixed with the starches. This digestive phase lasts for approximately thirty to forty-five minutes. However, if meat or other acid-forming foods, are added to this alkaline mixture, the splitting-down process of starches is stopped and these half-digested foods ferment in the stomach.

There have been a number of small scientific studies to support this theory. One early study carried out by three Philadelphia investigators in 1936 on five subjects revealed the levels of acidity in the stomach after protein meals, after starch meals, and after combined starch and protein meals. The results showed that, at one and a quarter hours after these meals were eaten, the stomach contents after the high protein meal were mostly acid; they were least acid after a high starch meal and they were halfway between the two states after a mixed meal. More significantly, the stomach contents after the combined meal revealed that the proteins were not being digested properly as the acid level was far lower than that required for an all-protein meal. The level of acidity had actually been reduced by two-thirds due to the presence of the starch foods. To put it simply, when starch and protein are eaten together, the alkaline components of the starch interfere with the digestion of the protein, and the acidity accompanying the protein foods likewise hinders the digestion of the starches.

This contrasts with the conventional theory that, when eating any kind of food, we produce gastric juices containing hydrochloric acid, and this destroys the alkaline medium. However, the Hay theory says that the protein present in carbohydrates, such as grains, is very small (about 10 percent) and is incomplete. Therefore, starches do not stimulate enough hydrochloric acid to interfere with the alkaline medium that is required for their digestion.

Nevertheless, many doctors today disagree with Dr Hay's explanation of the starch–protein theory and maintain that the gastric juice is necessary for the splitting of the starches. The starch is often contained in what are known as 'protein envelopes' which require the acid action so that the starch can be released. This is correct, but it does not alter the fact that the initial stage of starch digestion occurs in an alkaline medium for the first thirty minutes or so that it is in the stomach. After that, there is plenty of time for the gastric acid to digest the starches before they enter the small intestine. There, the pancreatic juice completes the digestion of carbohydrates and protein in a mostly alkaline medium. In the end, whichever theory is true does not really matter to the hundreds of thousands of people in Britain alone who have found that food combining works for them.

HEALTH BENEFITS

On first inspection, food combining may appear to be a frighteningly complicated eating regime in which the majority of traditional meals are banned. However, it is far more natural to eat in the way food combining dictates than to eat meals that contain all major food groups. Anthropological and archaeological evidence shows that our ancestors, the hunter–gatherers, had a healthy existence on a high-alkaline diet of berries, shoots, nuts and seeds (the gathered food) with occasional meat (the hunted food). The gathered food would have been eaten in its natural state and, although it would have been cooked, it would not have been served with potatoes and cabbage or tossed in some spaghetti! The stone-age diet was rich in fibre and fresh produce whereas today we clog our bodies with a combination of processed carbohydrates and proteins which are often high in sugar and saturated fat. It is not surprising our digestive system has trouble assimilating the resulting mess that ends up in the stomach. Today, we also eat far too many refined carbohydrates in the form of sugar, white bread, pasta and rice, too many of the wrong kinds of fat and not enough fibre and fresh produce. Food combining brings us closer to the natural diet of our forebears who, by all accounts, were far healthier and suffered far less from obesity and degenerative diseases than we do today. Advocates of food combining claim that it can help treat a variety of disorders including indigestion, constipation, obesity, diabetes mellitus, arthritis, allergies and skin conditions such as psoriasis and eczema. Ridding our body of toxins the food combining way can also help reduce cellulite and aid weight-loss.

FOOD GROUPS EXPLAINED

In order to combine foods successfully, we need to take a closer look at the different food groups: protein, carbohydrates, neutral foods, fruit and herbs and spices.

PROTEIN

Most of us are encouraged to believe that meat is a vital source of protein and without it, our bodies would be seriously lacking, but this is simply not true. In fact, we generally eat far more protein than our bodies need and we can easily obtain sufficient protein from a good mix of cereals and vegetables. Whether we eat protein in the form of meat, cereals or vegetables, it has to be broken down into the various amino acids, which are then reassembled to form human protein.

PROTEIN FOODS

Meat

We have all heard something about the recent scares surrounding factory-farmed meat, with B.S.E. having been particularly in the limelight. Factory-farmed animals are routinely fed growth hormones, antibiotics and other chemicals which only add to the burden of toxic waste inside us. The healthiest option is to buy organically-reared meat, although this is more expensive. Alternatively buy free-range poultry and lamb.

Fish

Fish is a healthier source of protein than meat. It contains less fat and the fat it does contain is of the beneficial, polyunsaturated kind. In fact, fish oil is extremely good for us and is an excellent source of vitamins A and D and essential fatty acids. It is best to buy fresh fish and cook it within twenty-four hours as some frozen fish is sprayed with chemical preservatives and this is not always declared on the label. Processed fish, ie salted and smoked, should also be kept to a minimum as processing destroys many of the nutrients that are present in fish in its natural state.

Eggs

Eggs are a rich source of protein but, like all animal products, they are also high in saturated fat. Always use free-range eggs as those from battery-reared hens may contain artificial colours and additives and, apart from anything else, free-range eggs taste better and involve far less appalling cruelty to the hens.

Cheese

All cheeses, no matter what animal they come from, are protein foods, although some cream cheese and cottage cheese contain very low levels of protein and can be mixed with carbohydrates, such as baked potatoes and bread.

Milk

In general, milk does not combine well with other foods and is also very mucus forming, which can cause trouble with our sinuses. Although milk is a complete source of protein and rich in calcium, many people are intolerant to cows' milk because the enzymes it contains are difficult to digest. When milk is mixed with other foods it is even more difficult to digest, as it interferes with the digestion of both proteins and carbohydrates. Those who are intolerant to cows' milk may find that they can cope better with goats' or sheeps' milk, but these should not be mixed with other foods either.

Soya milk is not really milk at all, but a white liquid made from soya beans. It does not taste like cows' milk but some do use it as a substitute. However, it is a processed product and the protein molecules in soya milk are very large, bigger than in cows' milk, and so some therapists warn it puts extra strain on our overworked digestive systems.

Yoghurt

Yoghurt is a great source of protein and it is easier to digest than milk. Choose the low-fat varieties which contain live cultures of the friendly bacteria. Although yoghurt is a protein, it can be mixed occasionally with oats to make muesli.

CARBOHYDRATES

Carbohydrates, or starches, provide the energy we need to carry out all our bodily processes. Starch foods include wheat and grains such as bread, pasta and rice and also some fruit and vegetables, such as potatoes and bananas. We need to eat these foods in order to get the energy we need, and some of us need more than others. For example, athletes need to eat plenty of carbohydrate to replenish the energy they burn off in exercise.

Wheat and other grains

Wheat is Britain's most important crop and, not surprisingly, our diet is dominated by it. Unfortunately, all wheat products such as bread and pasta have a high gluten content which many are sensitive to, causing symptoms such as diarrhoea, lethargy and skin disorders. However, it is possible to find wheat products which do not have such a high gluten content, such as rye bread. Much of the bread available from supermarkets also contains 'improvers' and other additives to keep the bread soft, and fresh-looking for longer. Look for brands such as Vogel which use organically-grown wheat and contain no additives.

Wheat bran

Wheat bran is *not* the best fibre provider and is, in fact, rough and difficult to digest. Wheat bran irritates the sensitive colon wall and often causes food intolerance and bowel disorders. This can result in poor elimination of waste – contrary to what most of us are led to believe.

Cracked wheat, or bulgar

This is a processed wheat product made from broken grains. The most nutritious way to eat cracked wheat is pre-soaked and it can be used to make a delicious salad dish called Tabbouleh (see page 89).

Semolina

This is the grittiest part of durum wheat, sifted out and made into hardened pasta products.

Wholewheat
This is from the wholewheat kernel and it is the best way to enjoy wheat.

Barley
Unrefined barley (pot barley) has high levels of iron, calcium, potassium and B vitamins (notably folic acid) and it can help to soothe the stomach, digestive and urinary tracts.

Buckwheat
Despite its name, buckwheat is totally gluten-free and nothing like our common wheat. It actually comes from a small plant related to rhubarb. Buckwheat contains B vitamins, potassium, magnesium and iron as well as the eight essential amino acids. Buckwheat grouts can be cooked in the same way as rice, and buckwheat flour can be used in baking recipes and to thicken sauces and soups.

Basmati rice
This is a fragrant Indian long-grain rice. It has a lovely aromatic flavour and brown basmati rice is best.

Brown rice
This is the entire rice pellet, including its protective bran coating, and is an excellent source of fibre. Brown rice also contains iron, calcium, B vitamins and many essential amino acids.

Maize
This is a versatile, gluten-free grain and can be eaten whole in the form of corn-on-the-cob, served as sweet corn or ground into cornflour.

Millet
This is not just budgie food, it is also a highly nutritious cereal and can be used as an alternative to rice. Before boiling, crack the seeds open by frying them in a little olive oil to allow them to absorb enough cooking water to become soft.

Oats
Oats are an important staple food and contain protein, B vitamins and even the healthy polyunsaturated fats. Porridge is an excellent energy-giving breakfast.

Rye
Rye has a similar composition to wheat but has a low gluten content. Many who find themselves allergic to wheat and its products, such as bread, can eat rye bread as an alternative.

Bananas and Potatoes

Both bananas and potatoes are at least 20 percent starch so they count as carbohydrate instead of neutral foods like other fruits and vegetables. This means you should not mix them with protein foods – so no more meat and potatoes! The best way to reap the nutritional benefits of potatoes is to eat them in their skins. Baked potatoes are very low in calories and make a tasty substantial meal with some butter and salad. Choose organic if possible, as the skins are not sprayed with anti-sprouting chemicals.

Pulses – A Food Combining Conundrum

Pulses (or legumes) include beans, lentils, peas, chickpeas and peanuts. They do not easily slot into the food combining jigsaw as they have high concentrations of both starch and protein. Dr Hay classified them as starch and thought that they were best avoided, but many beans are a rich source of protein which is important for vegetarians. Unfortunately, pulses do not mix well with carbohydrates or proteins and are renowned for causing flatulence, hence the jokes about baked beans. Soya beans and soya products such as tofu, tempeh, miso, soya flour and soya milk are all concentrated proteins and can cause digestive problems in some.

Sprouted pulses

By far the best way to eat pulses is when they are sprouted. This can easily be done at home, by soaking and then leaving the beans on a damp tea cloth on the window-sill or in an airing cupboard. Most grains, beans and seeds can be sprouted this way and it increases their vitamin, mineral and enzyme levels dramatically, as well as converting the starch into natural sugars. The most successful varieties of pulses for spouting are alfalfa, lentils and mung beans. They are delicious eaten raw in salads or simply sprinkled with a little freshly squeezed lemon juice. Sprouted pulses are neutral and can be mixed with both proteins and carbohydrates.

Sugar

As we have seen, refined sugar is one of the biggest dietary baddies, particularly refined white sugar. It does us absolutely no good whatsoever, and is linked to obesity and diabetes as well as a possible link to mental disturbances such as hyperactivity and even violent behaviour. Our consumption of refined sugar has increased dramatically since the 1960s with the huge variety of sweets, cakes and biscuits which are now available. Sugar is also added to most processed foods from baked beans to chicken curry, so look carefully on packaging to check for this.

NEUTRAL FOODS

The title 'neutral' means that these foods mix well with both carbohydrates and proteins and also combine well with each other.

Vegetables

Vegetables are a rich source of vitamins and minerals, high in fibre, low in calories and low in fat. Due to modern farming methods it is best to use organically grown vegetables which have not been sprayed with toxic pesticides, herbicides and fungicides. Much of the fruit and vegetables we get in the UK is imported and we have no idea of what chemicals are used in their cultivation. If you cannot get hold of organically grown fruit and vegetables, then make sure you either remove the skins or scrub them thoroughly with soapy water. Some, but not all of the chemical residues can be removed by thorough cleaning.

Nuts and seeds

Nuts are a highly concentrated food and should only be eaten in small amounts with starch and protein meals. They are a rich source of polyunsaturated oils which are very good for us healthwise, but are unfortunately high in calories. Always eat nuts slowly so that they can be broken up in the mouth where the process of digestion begins. Avoid processed nuts, ie salted or dry roasted varieties.

Seeds

Seeds are rich in vitamins, minerals and essential fatty acids. However, seeds turn rancid if not properly stored. They are best kept in an airtight container in the refrigerator. In general, seeds are easy to digest and are great to snack on.

Fats and Oils

Fats and oils are neutral so they can be used in both protein and carbohydrate meals. Cream is also neutral, but, due to its high levels of calories and saturated fat, should be avoided by those on the *Bikini Diet*!

FRUITS AND FRUIT JUICES

Fresh fruit and their juices are the easiest foods for our body to digest, assimilate and eliminate. In fact, an apple takes only about fifteen minutes to pass through the stomach, whereas a heavy protein meal will take at least five hours. Fruit is also a great fibre provider and contains a wealth of vitamins and minerals. It is 70 percent water, very low in calories and is ideal for flushing out the internal system and aiding weight-loss. With food combining, we should eat one totally alkaline meal a day and breakfast is often the best time for this. The majority of proteins and carbohydrates are all acid-forming – this means that their end products after digestion are acidic. With a few exceptions, only fruit, vegetables and yoghurt are alkaline. Up until midday our body is still in its elimination mode and eating fruit for breakfast will boost these processes. Fruit is also rich in enzymes which assists in its digestion. Some fruit, such as apples, also contain a substance called pectin which aids the removal of toxins.

However, it is not so good for us to eat fruit after a meal as a dessert. Fruit is designed to go straight through our digestive system and so it is best eaten on an empty stomach. It is then easily digested without using up any energy that may be needed to eliminate toxins and break down fat. If you eat an apple after a protein meal, the fruit will either speed up the passage of protein, which is then made to leave the stomach before it is properly digested, or the protein will cause the fruit to stay too long in the stomach so that it starts to ferment and turn to acid. Neither event is desirable as poorly digested protein and rotten fruit just add to our store of toxins and can cause indigestion pains.

Stewed fruit

Dr Hay believed that stewed fruits are 'dead fruits' and for optimum health we should be eating as much 'live' food as possible. Heat changes the chemical status of fruit, making it more acidic and destroying many of its important vitamins and enzymes.

Dried fruit

Dried fruits are also alkaline-forming and they mix well with each other, but should not be mixed with protein or starch. Most dried fruit is sprayed with glazing agents and sulphur dioxide preservatives and these are best avoided – so check on the packaging. You can buy additive-free dried fruit from health food stores. Raisins and dried apricots are great to snack on and they help to stimulate bowel movements.

HERBS AND SPICES

There are thousands of aromatic herbs and spices, such as basil, oregano, coriander and mint which add a great deal of flavour to our cooking. Herbs and spices are neutral and can be eaten in abundance with all foods, which is just as well considering how bland our meals would be without them. Herbs, when fresh, are packed with nutrients and have been used for centuries in cooking, in beauty therapies and to treat numerous ailments.

ACID OR ALKALINE?

Dr Hay believed that a balanced diet should consist of 25 percent acid-forming and 75 percent alkaline-forming food. Study the table below to see at a glance the foods that are alkaline-forming and those which are acid-forming:

ACID-FORMING FOOD

barley
beans
bread
breakfast cereals
buckwheat
cashew nuts
cheese
chickpeas
eggs
fish
flour
game
meat
oats
peas (dried)
peanuts
pecan nuts
poultry
rice
sugar
walnuts
wheat and wheat products

ALKALINE-FORMING FOOD

almonds
Brazil nuts
chestnuts
fruits
hazelnuts
millet
pine kernels
vegetables
yoghurt

PROTEIN OR CARBOHYDRATE?

Study the table below to discover at a glance which foods are protein, carbohydrate or neutral. The foods in the left column must <u>not</u> be mixed with the foods in the right column. The neutral foods in the central column can be mixed with the foods in both the left and right columns:

PROTEIN	NEUTRAL	CARBOHYDRATE
cheese	butter	biscuits
eggs	cream	bread
fish	herbs	cakes
meat	oil	crackers
milk	nuts	millet
poultry	salads	maize (corn)
shellfish	seeds	oats
soya beans	spreads	pasta
soya products	all vegetables except	pastry
	potatoes, sweet	
	potatoes and	
	Jerusalem artichokes	
yoghurt	all salads	potatoes
		rice
		sweet potatoes
		sugar
		honey
		maple syrup
		sweets
		sweet fruits such as custard apples, dates, figs, extra sweet grapes, papaya and pears (if very sweet and ripe)

YOUR SHOPPING LIST

It is a good idea to make sure that your cupboards and fridge are full of the fresh ingredients you need to make food combining easy. Apart from large amounts of fresh fruit and vegetables, there are other foods which are the basis for tasty, healthy meals. It is important to read all food labelling carefully to see what chemicals have been added to the food and choose organically grown food wherever possible and free-range chicken and eggs.

* brown rice
* extra virgin olive oil – the healthiest oil there is!
* free-range eggs
* dried fruit – raisins, sultanas and dried figs
  (these are all great for snacking on and for making fruit compôte)
* garlic and other herbs (preferably fresh), such as basil, bay leaves, coriander, fennel, oregano, parsley, peppermint, rosemary, tarragon and thyme
* black pepper and sea salt for seasoning
* oatbran, oatmeal or oatgerm
* nuts – Brazils, almonds, pecans, pinenuts and walnuts
* seeds – pumpkin seeds, sunflower seeds and linseeds
* soy or tamari sauce
* wholewheat bread
* wholegrain crackers
* wholewheat pasta
* cracked wheat
* free-range poultry
* fresh fish
* alternatives to ordinary table sugar: blackstrap molasses, organic unblended honey, natural maple syrup, fructose (fruit sugar which is useful for baking and it is twice as sweet as ordinary sugar and so half the amount is needed).

TIPS FOR SUCCESSFUL FOOD COMBINING

* Never mix concentrated proteins and carbohydrates
* Neutral foods can be mixed with both carbohydrates and proteins
* Use refined or cold-pressed vegetable oils such as sunflower, corn, olive, soya or wheatgerm, which are all high in polyunsaturates. Fry vegetables only very lightly in hot olive oil to preserve their goodness

* Always look for fresh, quality food when shopping, preferably organic, as this will contain less chemical pesticides and hormones than food which is farmed using modern methods
* Try to have more vegetables with each meal and cut down on concentrated starch and protein. For example, if you are having lamb chops and courgettes as a meal, limit yourself to one lamb chop, but go mad on the courgettes
* Avoid all refined and processed foods
* Try to fill up on your main meals so that you can leave a gap of four hours until you next eat something
* Cut down on the amount of salt you use in your cooking, and use only a pinch of sea salt
* Cut down on the amount of sugar you eat, and if you need something sweet use blackstrap molasses, honey, real maple syrup or crystallised ginger
* Instead of frying meat, poultry or fish, cook them gently in a covered pan in their own juices or roast them in the oven.

LOW-ENERGY FOODS

One of the aims of food combining is to cut out low-energy foods because they are not life-giving foods. Here, 'energy' does not refer to calories but to vitality value and, in fact, low-energy foods tend to be high in calories but can actually sap our energy if eaten in excess because the body finds them difficult to digest and metabolise, or they over-stimulate the system. Low-energy foods are:

* artificial sweeteners
* artificial colours, flavours and preservatives
* white and brown sugar
* sweets and chocolate
* coffee, tea, cocoa, cola, hot chocolate
* alcohol
* most polyunsaturated spreads
* processed 'low-fat' foods
* cows' milk and soya milk
* white flour and bread
* pizzas, pastries, pies and refined pasta
* salt
* salty snacks such as salted peanuts
* beef, pork and related products
* processed, smoked and coloured cheeses
* burned food
* deep-fried foods.

DRINKS

You do not need to worry about drinking small amounts of tea and coffee or combining them with other foods. However, if tea and coffee are drunk close to meal-times they can interfere with the absorption of certain nutrients. For example, if you drink tea or coffee up to half an hour after a meal, it will destroy much of the vitamin C gained from eating that meal. It is best to drink beverages in moderation in between meals. Herb teas are a great alternative to tea and coffee, which are both high in caffeine. Fizzy drinks are best avoided as they can fill the stomach with air and interfere with digestion.

Cows' milk and soya milk are both difficult to digest and some may wish to avoid milk altogether. Many people are intolerant to cows' milk (including my son Guy), and this can lead to the development of colds, diarrhoea, catarrh and other conditions which involve an excess of mucus. Nuts, seeds, pulses and many vegetables are good, alternative sources of calcium. Soya milk is often thought of as a healthy alternative to cows' milk, but it is a processed food which can also be difficult to digest. Rice milk is a good alternative (available from health shops).

WATER

Drinking water is extremely good for us as it helps to cleanse our digestive system and replenishes our water supplies. We should aim to drink six to eight glasses of still mineral water a day in addition to other drinks. However, we should not drink water with our meals as it dilutes the food and makes it pass too quickly through the system without being fully digested. Leave a gap of half an hour before and after meals before you drink water. Avoid tap water as it contains many unhealthy chemicals including nitrates, chlorine and aluminium. Either drink pure mineral water or buy a jug-style water filter which can sift out most of these undesirable substances. One of the best ways to cleanse your system morning and evening is to have a glass of hot water containing a slice of lemon. Lemon is a diuretic and it encourages the elimination of toxins.

ALCOHOL

Large amounts of alcohol should not be drunk as this will upset digestion, but to drink alcohol in moderation is fine – follow the guidelines on page 19. Drinking wine with your meal should not interfere with its digestion as long as you drink in moderation, so don't worry about combining alcohol with foods.

JUICES

Fresh juices have the power to nourish, cleanse, protect, soothe and heal. They are nutritious and easy to digest and give us energy in a naturally delicious drink. Most cartons of juice will contain additives and preservatives, so it is best to make your own juices with an electric juicer or blender. In addition, processed fruit juices turn acidic after lengthy exposure to the atmosphere. Juices are much more than just a drink, they are meals in themselves and one fresh juice will have more nutritional value than most of the processed meals available from supermarkets. It makes sense, then, to drink fresh juices every day. They are a delicious and refreshing way to reap all the nutritious benefits of fruit and vegetables and there are endless combinations. To make your own juices, invest in a high-speed electric juicer, available from department stores at around £35. The best fruit and vegetables for boosting the digestive system are: beetroot, carrot, celery, cucumber, endive, grapefruit, lemon, papaya, pear, pineapple, radish, raspberry and watercress, so get juicing! For more information about the health benefits of juicing and great juice recipes read my book Juicing (Boxtree, £3.99).

For more information about food combining see *Liz Earle's Quick Guide to Food Combining* (Boxtree, £3.99).

Section 4

GO!

The *Bikini Diet* gives you six weeks of original and interesting menu plans. **You should strictly follow the *Bikini Diet* menus for at least six weeks to lose a stone.**

All the recipes for the *Bikini Diet* are tasty and nutritious. They use colourful seasonal fruits and vegetables and are a treat to look at as well as to eat. Many of the recipe ideas were inspired by my favourite summer holiday hot spots, including Spain, Greece, Turkey, Indonesia and the Caribbean. So even if you're planning to stay at home this year, you can still enjoy a taste of the exotic!

The problem with most diets is that they are very boring. We soon feel deprived and unhappy (and this is the main reason why most diets don't work). The *Bikini Diet* makes it possible to slim while still enjoying good food. I have included as many varied recipes as will fit into this book. There are lots of new ideas to tempt the taste-buds and make eating feel like a treat and not an endurance test. A few recipes use new and unusual ingredients that you may not have come across before. In some cases, you may have to hunt out the ingredients in larger supermarkets or delicatessens. I have also included a few stockists in Useful Addresses at the back of the book to help track down the more unusual items. But don't worry if you can't find a particular ingredient. You can always leave it out or use your imagination for a substitute. Most of the recipes are simple to prepare, but there is also a range of *Bikini Diet* Instant Options starting on page 70 for when you don't have time to cook.

When writing a menu plan it is impossible to please everyone all the time. However, I have tried to make the meals as interesting and practical as possible, with plenty of vegetarian options and ideas for eating with friends. When following the *Bikini Diet* menu plans, keep in mind the following important points:

* The meals for each day are calorie counted to total around 1,200Kcals or less.
* If you are too busy to cook any dish, or need something practical to take to work as a packed lunch, follow the *Bikini Diet* Instant Options on page 70. These are quick and easy alternatives to the more interesting recipes and can be substituted for lunch or supper. Always make sure your daily calorie allowance is 1,200Kcals or less.
* Some of the menu plans are lower in calories than others. This is to help fool the metabolism. If you stick to a very low-calorie diet the

body may see it as a famine situation and lower the metabolism to protect itself. Varying your calorie intake helps prevent this. On days with a lower calorie intake there is a little leeway left for treats, such as a few squares of chocolate or an ice-cream if the weather's hot. Use your judgement though, and take care not to undo all your good work!

* Unless the recipe says it serves one always measure your meals. Get to know what each calorie-counted portion looks like. When in doubt, get the scales out.

* If you're cooking for one, reduce the quantities in the recipes accordingly and, when possible, store any leftover portions in the freezer. Clearly label each pot or bag so you can easily identify the contents. Try not to keep spare meals in the fridge which you may be tempted to nibble on.

* Many of the recipes use small amounts of olive oil as it is monounsaturated and has a good flavour. But it is fine to use sunflower, safflower or other cheaper blended cooking oils instead.

* Always use low-fat versions where possible – such as low-fat yoghurts, fromage frais, cottage cheese, etc. These really do reduce your calories and fat-grams without sacrificing taste. Look for low-fat 'live' or 'bio' yoghurts as these contain friendly bacteria which are good for the digestive system and can improve our health.

* The *Bikini Diet* menu plans include a snack for each weekday. This is to help ward off hunger pangs while you're at work or home looking after the kids. The weekend menu plans feature a few more adventurous meals that are good for family meals or for entertaining a few friends without breaking your diet!

* The *Bikini Diet* is designed to be followed for at least six weeks. You can follow the menu plans for as long as you like to continue with your successful weight-loss.

* Make friends with food instead of thinking of it as the enemy. Take a few seconds to garnish a dish or arrange it attractively on the plate before serving – even if you're on your own. We eat with our eyes as well as our mouths, so use colourful ingredients and think about the presentation of each meal.

Food Combining Options

Many of the recipes in the menu plans follow the rules of food combining, but the plans are not designed for strict food combiners. However, there are three food combining days in each week of the menu plans provided you choose a food combining breakfast option. If you would like to keep rigidly to the rules of food combining, only follow the food combining recipes – those marked FC. These recipes are also labelled either P for Protein, C for Carbohydrate, or N for Neutral. Remember that you should never mix protein with carbohydrate and allow four hours between meals of different character. An additional aim of food combining is to eat a totally alkaline meal each day. The easiest way to achieve this is to eat a simple breakfast of fresh summer fruits and yoghurt, then a protein or a starch meal for lunch and supper (ie starch and then protein or protein and then starch – not two meals of the same character). If you need to snack, then have neutral foods such as fruit, nuts and seeds. If you are having a dessert make sure that it is the same character as the main meal, ie a carbohydrate meal should be followed by a carbohydrate dessert. Don't worry if you find this eating regime too strict, as it is important that you can relax and enjoy your food. If you have a bad day, then you can make up for it the next day. For any diet to work, it is important to set yourself easily achievable goals.

Food Combining Sandwich Fillings

Many traditional recipes are not allowed on the food combining diet and most common sandwich fillings are also banned as they combine starch (bread) with protein (tuna, ham, egg, cheese etc.) However, there are many delicious, healthy alternatives to these fillings to choose from below:

* Mixed sliced vegetables with fresh herbs
* Sliced cucumber and cress
* Nut Butter (see recipe on page 127)
* Cottage cheese with chopped chives
* Mashed banana
* Dates and chopped celery
* Avocado and Alfalfa (see recipe on page 76)
* Tahini and Cucumber (see recipe on page 90)

Vegetarian options

Most of the *Bikini Diet* recipes are suitable for vegetarians, as this is the healthiest way of eating. However, there are still plenty of meat and fish recipes for those who want them. Vegetarians will be able to adapt many of these by using meat substitutes, such as Quorn and tofu. In some cases I give a vegetarian alternative to a meat or fish recipe. Most of the recipes rely on healthy, low-fat ingredients such as fruits, vegetables and wholegrains such as rice and pasta.

A word about drinks

As mentioned in Section 1, you can have a small weekly alcohol allowance while following the *Bikini Diet*. This is as follows:

* three small glasses of red, white or rosé wine *or*
* three half-pints of lager *or*
* three single measures of spirits with optional low-calorie mixers, such as diet tonic water or ginger ale.

You are also allowed up to four cups of tea or coffee a day. This can either be normal or decaffeinated. It is best to drink these black, but if you can't bear the taste add a splash of semi-skimmed or skimmed milk. Avoid cappuccino coffee as this is high in fat. Use sweeteners instead of sugar, but try to get used to drinking tea or coffee unsweetened. In addition, you may also drink as many cups of herb or fruit teas as you fancy. You can also have up to two diet drinks a day (such as diet colas, lemonade, etc.) but the best option is to drink plenty of water. It's important to keep your fluid intake high, especially during the hotter summer months. Try to drink four–six large glasses of water a day. I keep a 1.5 litre bottle of mineral water on my desk and try to finish it every day.

Portion control

It is important to measure the portions of food for this eating plan to be successful. When in doubt – don't guess – get out the scales. This will ensure that you eat only the quantity allowed and is also a useful way of learning exactly what a calorie-counted portion of food looks like.

The following is a guideline to the portions used throughout the *Bikini Diet* weekly menu plans.

Bread – 1 portion = 1 medium wholemeal slice
Rice – 1 portion = 4 tbsp cooked brown rice
Rolls – 1 portion = 1 small wholemeal roll with 1tsp low-fat spread
New potatoes – 1 portion = 150g (6oz) boiled, with skins
Vegetables – 1 portion = 100g (4oz) mixed vegetables, such as carrots, broccoli, leeks, cauliflower, peas and green beans
Mixed salad – 1 portion = 100g (4oz) lettuce, tomatoes, peppers, carrots, spring onions, watercress, cucumber, etc.
Green salad – 1 portion = 100g (4oz) mixed lettuces, e.g. batavia, little gem, endive, frisée, lamb's lettuce, etc.
Pulses – 1 portion = 100g (4oz) cooked lentils, chickpeas, kidney beans, butter beans, etc.
Juice – 1 portion = 150ml (5fl oz) or medium-sized glass

BIKINI DIET
BREAKFAST CHOICES

It's important not to skip breakfast. Missing breakfast leads to a severe drop in blood sugar levels mid-morning, making us more likely to snap at those around us and reach for the biscuits or chocolate bars. Choose from the following selection each morning – every option is quick and simple so won't take much time to make. Each option contains an average of 170Kcals, except for the Wake-up Shake which is 260 Kcals.

Option 1
Fruit Compôte – see recipe on page 74. FC (P)

Option 2
Summer Muesli – see recipe on page 74.

Option 3
Low-sugar cereal – one 30g (1¼oz) serving with 125ml (4fl oz) semi-skimmed milk. Choose from Rice Krispies, Weetabix, Kallo Puffed Rice Cereal, Special K or Puffed Kashi (mixed grains, from health-food shops). Serve with 50g (2oz) chopped strawberries (optional).

Option 4
Juice and toast – one slice of medium wholemeal bread, toasted, with 1tsp low-fat spread. Served with one medium glass of apple or orange juice. FC (C)

Option 5
Wake-up Shake – see recipe on page 75. FC (N)

Plus
One cup of tea or coffee from your daily drink allowance.

BIKINI DIET MENU PLANS

Week 1

Day	Menu	Page	Kcals
Monday			
Breakfast	*Bikini Diet* breakfast choice	(page 57)	170
Lunch	Tuna-stuffed pitta pocket	(page 93)	294
	Mixed salad with 2 tsp low-calorie vinaigrette		35
	1 large orange		80
Evening	Vegetable stir-fry with cashew nuts and rice noodles	(page 100)	253
	Pot of low-fat yoghurt		55
Snack	1 banana		100
	75g (3oz) raisins		246
Total Kcals			*1233*
Tuesday			
Breakfast	*Bikini Diet* breakfast choice	(page 57)	170
Lunch	Tahini and cucumber sandwich	(page 90)	165
	1 banana		100
Evening	Halibut with watercress sauce	(page 118)	434
	Portion of vegetables		60
	Rippled fruit fool	(page 134)	127
Snack	1 large apple		80
	Pot of low-fat yoghurt		55
Total Kcals			*1191*
Wednesday			
Breakfast	*Bikini Diet* breakfast choice	(page 57)	170
Lunch	Spanish omelette	(page 87)	205
	Low-calorie Tricolore	(page 82)	148
Evening	Cabbage parcels	(page 90)	190
	Portion of vegetables		60
	Spiced bananas	(page 135)	198
Snack	4 average breadsticks		60
	40g (1¾oz) dried prunes		100
Total Kcals			*1156*

Thursday

Breakfast	*Bikini Diet* breakfast choice	(page 57)	170
Lunch	Low-fat chicken liver pâté	(page 82)	145
	3 rice cakes with 2 tsp low-fat spread		138
	Carrot and celery sticks		30
	3 fresh figs		111
Evening	Warm seafood and pasta salad	(page 126)	365
	Half a mango or 100g (4oz) grapes		68
Snack	2 *Bikini Diet* brownies	(page 130)	152
Total Kcals			*1179*

Friday

Breakfast	*Bikini Diet* breakfast choice	(page 57)	170
Lunch	Baked potato with creamy cottage cheese	(page 71)	275
	Mixed salad with 2 tsp low-calorie vinaigrette dressing		35
Evening	Lemon chicken	(page 105)	300
	2 portions of mixed vegetables		120
	Pot of low-fat yoghurt		55
Snack	1 large orange		80
	1 large apple		80
Total Kcals			*1115*

Saturday

Breakfast	*Bikini Diet* breakfast choice	(page 57)	170
Lunch	Ratatouille and pasta salad		260
	1 wholemeal pitta bread		159
Evening	Halibut with watercress sauce	(page 118)	434
	Portion of new potatoes		123
	Portion of vegetables		60
Snack	Rippled fruit fool	(page 134)	127
Total Kcals			*1333*

Sunday

Breakfast	*Bikini Diet* breakfast choice	(page 57)	170
Lunch	Chicken stuffed with spinach and cheese	(page 76)	305
	Baked potato with 1 tsp low-fat yoghurt		225
	2 kiwi fruit		89
Evening	Basmati vegetable pilaf	(page 65)	233
Snack	Mandarin jelly	(page 133)	226
Total Kcals			*1248*

Week 1 – Analysis of Dishes

Vegetarian	Six
Fish	Four
Meat	Three

Food Combining Days

Tuesday
Wednesday
Friday

Week 2

Day	Menu	Page	Kcals
Monday			
Breakfast	*Bikini Diet* breakfast choice	(page 57)	170
Lunch	Warm goat's cheese salad	(page 94)	214
	Small wholemeal roll with 1tsp low-fat spread		160
	1 nectarine		67
Evening	Prawn kebabs with herb dressing	(page 121)	287
	Portion of rice		127
	Portion of vegetables		60
Snack	Pot of St Michael Lite toffee mousse, or similar		91
	1 plum		36
Total Kcals			*1212*
Tuesday			
Breakfast	*Bikini Diet* breakfast choice	(page 57)	170
Lunch	Low-fat hummous	(page 83)	182
	2 wholemeal pitta breads		318
	Pot of diet fromage frais		50
	2 fresh figs		74
Evening	Wild mushroom risotto	(page 100)	164
	Strawberry chinchilla with an orange sauce	(page 135)	199
Snack	100g (4oz) strawberries		34
Total Kcals			*1191*
Wednesday			
Breakfast	*Bikini Diet* breakfast choice	(page 57)	170
Lunch	Baked potato with 1tsp low-fat spread		236
	Tabbouleh	(page 89)	188
	1 banana		100
Evening	Spiced prawns	(page 123)	268
	Portion of vegetables		60
	150g (5oz) of cherries		104
Snack	Pot of low-fat yoghurt		55
Total Kcals			*1181*
Thursday			
Breakfast	*Bikini Diet* breakfast choice	(page 57)	170
Lunch	Lean pork chop, grilled		280
	Raw apple sauce	(page 127)	54
	Portion of vegetables		60
	Portion of rice		127
	1 large orange		80

Evening	Thai marinaded chicken and vegetable kebabs	(page 113)	247
	40g (1¾oz) dried prunes		100
Snack	Pot of low-fat chocolate dessert		60
Total Kcals			*1178*

Friday

Breakfast	*Bikini Diet* breakfast choice	(page 57)	170
Lunch	Cottage cheese and summer fruits platter	(page 71)	103
	2 wholemeal pitta breads, sliced		318
	1 banana		100
Evening	Chicken with peppers	(page 103)	417
	Portion of vegetables		60
Snack	1 large apple		80
Total Kcals			*1248*

Saturday

Breakfast	*Bikini Diet* breakfast choice	(page 57)	170
Lunch	Sunshine salad	(page 89)	240
	Small wholemeal roll with 1tsp low-fat spread		160
Evening	Lamb paprika	(page 57)	256
	2 portions of vegetables		120
	Mandarin jelly	(page 133)	226
Snack	Snack pot of low-fat yoghurt		55
Total Kcals			*1227*

Sunday

Breakfast	*Bikini Diet* breakfast choice	(page 57)	170
Lunch	Greek spring salad	(page 79)	190
	2 thin slices of pumpernickel bread with 2 tsp low-fat spread		193
	Pot of low-fat chocolate dessert		60
Evening	Fillets of sole with pink grapefruit and lime	(page 116)	358
	Black cherry clafouti	(page 130)	183
Snack	1 large apple		80
Total Kcals			*1234*

Week 2 – Analysis of Dishes		**Food Combining Days**
Vegetarian	Seven	Wednesday
Fish	Three	Friday
Meat	Four	Saturday

Week 3

Day	Menu	Page	Kcals
Monday			
Breakfast	*Bikini Diet* breakfast choice	(page 57)	170
Lunch	Tomato and vegetable soup	(page 91)	23
	Endive and apple salad	(page 78)	173
	Small wholemeal roll with 1tsp low-fat spread		160
	1 banana		100
Evening	Thai marinaded chicken and vegetable kebabs	(page 113)	247
	Portion of vegetables		60
	Pot of low-fat yoghurt		55
Snack	Mandarin jelly	(page 133)	226
Total Kcals			*1214*

Day	Menu	Page	Kcals
Tuesday			
Breakfast	*Bikini Diet* breakfast choice	(page 57)	170
Lunch	Cottage cheese and summer fruits platter	(page 71)	103
	2 wholemeal pitta breads		318
	1 banana		100
Evening	Tomato and vegetable soup	(page 91)	23
	Fast fish risotto	(page 114)	290
	Portion of vegetables		60
Snack	2 *Bikini Diet* brownies	(page 130)	152
Total Kcals			*1216*

Day	Menu	Page	Kcals
Wednesday			
Breakfast	*Bikini Diet* breakfast choice	(page 57)	170
Lunch	Salmon with watercress sauce	(page 122)	243
	Portion of vegetables		60
	1 orange		80
	Pot of low-fat yoghurt		55
Evening	Buckwheat bonanza	(page 95)	250
	Courgette and carrot cake	(page 131)	226
Snack	1 banana		100
Total Kcals			*1184*

Day	Menu	Page	Kcals
Thursday			
Breakfast	*Bikini Diet* breakfast choice	(page 57)	170
Lunch	Baked potato with cucumber dressing	(page 71)	197
	Small wholemeal roll with 1tsp low-fat spread		160
	75g (3oz) sultanas		248
Evening	Spinach and macaroni pie	(page 99)	245

	Rippled fruit fool	(page 134)	127
Snack	1 large orange		80
Total Kcals			*1227*

Friday

Breakfast	*Bikini Diet* breakfast choice	(page 57)	170
Lunch	Tropical fish salad with a hot mango dressing	(page 92)	395
Evening	Stuffed mushrooms with hummous and fresh herbs	(page 99)	529
	Mixed salad with 2 tsp low-calorie vinaigrette		35
Snack	1 banana		100
Total Kcals			*1229*

Saturday

Breakfast	*Bikini Diet* breakfast choice	(page 57)	170
Lunch	Red pepper with tagliatelle and vegetables	(page 85)	186
	1 wholemeal pitta		159
	1 banana		100
Evening	Grilled salmon steaks with fennel	(page 117)	315
	Portion of vegetables		60
	Summer strawberries in a raspberry and passion-fruit sauce	(page 136)	134
Snack	1 apple		80
Total Kcals			*1204*

Sunday

Breakfast	*Bikini Diet* breakfast choice	(page 57)	170
Lunch	Stuffed Mediterranean tomatoes	(page 88)	170
	Small wholemeal roll with 1tsp low-fat spread		160
	Pot of low-fat yoghurt		55
Evening	Nasi Goreng (Indonesian pork and prawn rice)	(page 119)	521
	1 plum		36
Snack	1 apple		80
Total Kcals			*1192*

Week 3 – Analysis of Dishes

Vegetarian	Eight
Fish	Four
Meat	Two

Food Combining Days

Monday
Wednesday
Saturday

Week 4

Day	Menu	Page	Kcals
Monday			
Breakfast	*Bikini Diet* breakfast choice	(page 57)	170
Lunch	Mackerel fillets	(page 83)	409
	Portion of vegetables		60
Evening	Ratatouille and pasta salad	(page 85)	260
	Spiced bananas	(page 135)	198
Snack	1 wholemeal pitta bread		159
Total Kcals			*1256*
Tuesday			
Breakfast	*Bikini Diet* breakfast choice	(page 57)	170
Lunch	Spinach and prosciutto salad	(page 88)	109
	1 wholemeal pitta bread, warmed		159
	1 banana		100
Evening	Jamaica spiced cod with a tomato and coriander salsa	(page 118)	412
	Strawberry chinchilla with an orange sauce	(page 135)	199
Snack	Pot of low-fat yoghurt		55
Total Kcals			*1204*
Wednesday			
Breakfast	*Bikini Diet* breakfast choice	(page 57)	170
Lunch	Avocado and alfalfa sandwich	(page 76)	220
	Tabbouleh	(page 89)	188
	1 large orange		80
Evening	Five vegetable terrine	(page 97)	120
	Warm goat's cheese salad	(page 94)	214
	Rippled fruit fool	(page 134)	127
Snack	5 dried dates		114
Total Kcals			*1233*
Thursday			
Breakfast	*Bikini Diet* breakfast choice	(page 57)	170
Lunch	Tomato and feta cheese salad	(page 91)	235
	Small wholemeal roll with 1tsp low-fat spread		160
	Pot of low-fat yoghurt		55
Evening	*Sopa de Picadillo*	(page 108)	306
	Portion of vegetables		60
	Summer strawberries in a raspberry and passion-fruit sauce	(page 136)	134
Snack	1 banana		100
Total Kcals			*1220*

Friday

Breakfast	*Bikini Diet* breakfast choice	(page57)	170
Lunch	Roast vegetable kebabs with nutty rice	(page 86)	239
	1 large banana		100
Evening	Lemon chicken	(page 105)	300
	Herbed mushrooms	(page 81)	220
Snack	1 pear		98
Total Kcals			*1127*

Saturday

Breakfast	*Bikini Diet* breakfast choice	(page 57)	170
Lunch	Potato, bean and pepperoni salad	(page 85)	185
	1 wholemeal pitta bread		159
	Pot of Sainsbury's low-fat fool or similar		91
Evening	Risotto-stuffed aubergines with a spicy tomato sauce	(page 98)	379
	Green salad with 2 tbsp low-calorie vinaigrette dressing		24
	Summer strawberries in a raspberry and passion-fruit sauce	(page 136)	134
Snack	1 banana		100
Total Kcals			*1218*

Sunday

Breakfast	*Bikini Diet* breakfast choice	(page 57)	170
Lunch	Chilled melon with Parma ham and strawberry salsa	(page 77)	190
	Small wholemeal roll with 1tsp low-fat spread		160
	Pot of low-fat yoghurt		55
Evening	Thai chicken with prawn soup	(page 112)	259
	Mandarin jelly	(page 133)	226
	1 fresh fig		37
Snack	1 banana		100
Total Kcals			*1197*

Week 4 – Analysis of Dishes		**Food Combining Days**
Vegetarian	Six	Monday
Fish	Two	Wednesday
Meat	Six	Friday

Week 5

Day	Menu	Page	Kcals
Monday			
Breakfast	*Bikini Diet* breakfast choice	(page 57)	170
Lunch	No-cook rissoles	(page 83)	449
	Mixed salad with 2 tsp low-calorie vinaigrette		35
Evening	Lamb paprika	(page 104)	256
	Portion of vegetables		60
	Rippled fruit fool	(page 134)	127
Snack	1 large apple		80
Total Kcals			*1177*
Tuesday			
Breakfast	*Bikini Diet* breakfast choice	(page 57)	170
Lunch	Fishy jacket potatoes	(page 117)	279
	Green salad with 2 tsp low-calorie vinaigrette		25
	Pot of low-fat chocolate dessert		60
Evening	Pork and pasta stir-fry	(page 107)	246
	Black cherry clafouti	(page 130)	183
Snack	75g (3oz) raisins		246
Total Kcals			*1209*
Wednesday			
Breakfast	*Bikini Diet* breakfast choice	(page 57)	170
Lunch	Tomato and feta cheese salad	(page 91)	235
	Pot of low-fat yoghurt		55
	1 large orange		80
Evening	Vegetable stir-fry with cashew nuts	(page 100)	253
	Courgette and carrot cake	(page 131)	226
Snack	1 banana		100
Total Kcals			*1119*
Thursday			
Breakfast	*Bikini Diet* breakfast choice	(page 57)	170
Lunch	Pitta bread salad	(page 84)	510
Evening	Cod kebabs with basil sauce	(page 114)	333
	Portion of vegetables		60
	Mango ice cream	(page 133)	103
Total Kcals			*1176*

Friday
Breakfast	*Bikini Diet* breakfast choice	(page 57)	170
Lunch	Warm cod salad	(page 125)	164
	Great green salad	(page 79)	36
	Small wholemeal roll with 1tsp low-fat spread		160
Evening	Summer lamb hotpot	(page 111)	460
	Portion of rice		125
	Mango ice cream	(page 133)	103
Total Kcals			*1218*

Saturday
Breakfast	*Bikini Diet* breakfast choice	(page 57)	170
Lunch	Spicy rubbed chicken	(page109)	126
	Large baked potato		127
	Portion of vegetables		60
	Pot of low-fat yoghurt		55
Evening	Nasi Goreng (Indonesian pork and prawn rice)	(page 119)	521
	1 nectarine		67
Snack	2 fresh figs		74
Total Kcals			*1200*

Sunday
Breakfast	*Bikini Diet* breakfast choice	(page 57)	170
Lunch	Smoked mackerel, pasta and apple salad	(page 87)	371
	Pot of low-fat yoghurt		55
Evening	Lamb and bean ragout	(page 104)	237
	Portion of new potatoes		123
	Portion of vegetables		60
	Strawberry chinchilla with an orange sauce	(page 135)	199
Total Kcals			*1215*

Week 5 – Analysis of Dishes

Vegetarian	Four
Fish	Four
Meat	Six

Food Combining Days

Monday
Wednesday
Thursday

Week 6

Day Monday	Menu	Page	Kcals
Breakfast	*Bikini Diet* breakfast choice	(page 57)	170
Lunch	Spanish omelette	(page 87)	205
	1 wholemeal pitta bread		159
	Green salad with 2 tsp low-calorie vinaigrette dressing		25
Evening	Cod kebabs with basil sauce	(page 114)	333
	Portion of new potatoes		123
	Portion of vegetables		60
	1 banana		100
Snack	1 plum		36
Total Kcals			*1211*

Tuesday

Breakfast	*Bikini Diet* breakfast choice	(page 57)	170
Lunch	Asparagus and Parmesan salad	(page 75)	180
	Small wholemeal roll with 1tsp low-fat spread		160
	2 kiwi fruits		89
Evening	Spiced prawns	(page 123)	268
	Portion of rice		127
	Portion of vegetables		60
	Pot of low-fat yoghurt		55
Snack	Half a mango or 100g (4oz) of grapes		68
	1 plum		36
Total Kcals			*1213*

Wednesday

Breakfast	*Bikini Diet* breakfast choice	(page 57)	170
Lunch	Tabbouleh	(page 89)	188
	1 wholemeal pitta bread		159
	1 banana		100
Evening	Grilled salmon steaks with fennel	(page 117)	315
	Portion of vegetables		60
	Rippled fruit fool	(page 134)	127
Snack	1 large orange		80
Total Kcals			*1199*

Thursday

Breakfast	*Bikini Diet* breakfast choice	(page 57)	170
Lunch	Warm goat's cheese salad	(page 94)	214
	Pot of low-fat yoghurt		55
	1 large apple		80

Evening	Risotto-stuffed aubergines with		
	spicy tomato sauce	(page 98)	379
	1 wholemeal pitta bread		159
	Summer strawberries in a raspberry and		
	passion-fruit sauce	(page 136)	134
Total Kcals			*1191*

Friday

Breakfast	*Bikini Diet* breakfast choice	(page 57)	170
Lunch	Lean pork chop, grilled		280
	Raw apple sauce	(page 127)	54
	Portion of vegetables		60
	Portion of rice		127
	1 large orange		80
Evening	Tuna and sweetcorn potato cakes	(page 124)	237
	100g (4oz) low-calorie baked beans		73
	Rippled fruit fool	(page 134)	127
Total Kcals			*1205*

Saturday

Breakfast	*Bikini Diet* breakfast choice	(page 57)	170
Lunch	Roast vegetable kebabs with nutty rice	(page 86)	239
Evening	Chicken with peppers	(page 103)	417
	Portion of vegetables		60
	Mandarin jelly	(page 133)	226
Snack	1 large apple		80
Total Kcals			*1192*

Sunday

Breakfast	*Bikini Diet* breakfast choice	(page 57)	170
Lunch	Mild lamb korma	(page 106)	241
	Portion of rice		127
	Carrots and celery sticks		30
Evening	Chicken and pasta shell salad	(page 102)	244
	1 wholemeal pitta bread		159
	Black cherry clafouti	(page 130)	183
Snack	Pot of low-fat yoghurt		55
Total Kcals			*1209*

Week 6 – Analysis of Dishes

		Food Combining Days
Vegetarian	Six	Wednesday
Fish	Four	Thursday
Meat	Four	Saturday

BIKINI DIET
INSTANT OPTIONS

These are ideas for when time is tight, you need to take a packed lunch to work or you're just too tired to cook! Read through these recipes and keep a stock of ingredients at hand in your cupboard. Good time-savers are low-calorie baked beans, tinned tomatoes, precooked tinned rice, bottled passata (sieved tomatoes), baking potatoes and cottage cheese. Dried herbs and spices store for months on end, so keep a selection ready to liven up a simple quick-cook dish.

Tzatziki FC (P)

Serves 1	
Kcals	351
Fat	3.2g
Fibre	1.8g

This simple Greek meal is the perfect summer lunch. Use an empty yoghurt pot or small plastic container for a packed lunch.

Add 1 crushed clove of garlic (or teaspoon of garlic sauce) to 50g (2oz) low-fat Greek yoghurt. Stir in 2 tbsp grated cucumber. Season with a pinch of salt and pepper. Serve with two wholemeal pitta breads, cut into strips, or a neutral salad if you are food combining.

Golden Rice Salad FC (C)

Serves 1	
Kcals	247
Fat	1.6g
Fibre	4.5g

This is a good way to use up cold rice (always cook more than you need). Put 100g (4oz) cooked rice in a bowl. Add 2 tbsp tinned sweetcorn, 1 tbsp chopped cucumber, one large chopped tomato and a pinch of dried mixed herbs. Add 2 tbsp mango chutney, stir well and serve with a plain green salad.

Summer Stir-fry FC (N)

Serves 1	
Kcals	244
Fat	1.7g
Fibre	7.1g

Finely shred 50g (2oz) red cabbage, two large carrots, one courgette, one onion and half a fennel (or any other combination of ingredients you happen to have). Heat 1tsp oil in a wok or large saucepan and stir in the vegetables. Add a few drops of water to prevent burning (the steam this creates helps to cook the vegetables). Add a dash of tamari or soya sauce, a sprinkling of sesame seeds and serve.

Low-fat Instant Risotto FC (C)
Serves 1

Kcals   148
Fat   1.1g
Fibre   3.8g

Heat a few tablespoons of stock or water in the bottom of a wok or large pan. Add a chopped onion and cook until soft. Add 100g (4oz) cooked brown rice, 2 tbsp passata (sieved tomatoes), 1tsp dried basil and 1tbsp crushed garlic or garlic sauce. Stir and serve.

Cottage Cheese and Summer Fruits Platter FC (N)
Serves 1

Kcals   103
Fat   1.4g
Fibre   1.7g

Place 100g (4oz) low-fat cottage cheese (plain or with added flavourings) in the centre of a plate. Arrange 100g (4oz) mixed fruits around the outside. Good fruits to choose include melon slices, strawberries and grapes.

Baked Potatoes
The humble baked potato is the perfect choice for a hot, filling instant meal. I keep part-cooked baking potatoes in the fridge and crisp them up in a hot oven before eating with the following fillings.

Each recipe idea serves 1

Creamy Cottage Cheese FC (C)
Kcals   275
Fat   1.2g
Fibre   5.0g

Combine 100g (4oz) low-fat cottage cheese with 2 tbsp low-fat yoghurt, 1tsp garlic sauce and 1tsp dried herbs. Mix well and serve.

Yoghurt and Chive Dressing
Kcals   217
Fat   0.9g
Fibre   5.1g

See recipe on page 129. I keep this dressing handy in the fridge, ready for using. Use 2 tbsp on baked potatoes or for jazzing up a bowlful of leftover rice.

Cucumber Dressing
Kcals   197
Fat   0.4g
Fibre   5.5g

See recipe on page 128. This is another dressing I regularly make. It has a rich, almost creamy flavour even though it contains very little fat. Use 2 tbsp on a baked potato.

Orange and Tamari Dressing FC (C)

Kcals	205
Fat	0.4g
Fibre	5.5g

See recipe on page 128. This dressing has an unusually tangy flavour and is especially good on baked potatoes. Use 2 tbsp per portion.

No-cook Time Saver

Kcals	320
Fat	2.7g
Fibre	4.4g

If I'm travelling or filming on location I take this lunch-box with me. It's just a small wholemeal roll with 1tsp low-fat spread and a little Marmite, a banana and a small pot of low-fat fruit yoghurt. There's not many calories or fat-grams here, but plenty of fibre, calcium and vitamins.

Tomatoes on Toast FC (C)

Kcals	260
Fat	3.7g
Fibre	2.5g

Simply toast two slices of Vogel mixed grain brown bread and serve topped with 100g (4oz) tinned tomatoes. What could be easier? Vogel bread is tastier than most and also has almost half the fat of regular wholemeal.

Rice Cakes FC (C)

Kcals	238
Fat	5.0g
Fibre	3.0g

When there's no time at all, I simply spread 2 tsp low-fat spread and a dab of Marmite on to four crunchy rice cakes, topped with slices from one banana.

BIKINI DIET DESSERTS

The *Bikini Diet* includes low-fat, calorie-counted yoghurts and slimmer's desserts in the menu plans because they are easy to eat and generally taste good. Many are flavoured with chocolate or toffee, so can satisfy a sweet tooth without piling on the pounds. However, most do contain artificial additives, such as chemical sweeteners and sometimes synthetic flavourings too. Before buying, read the labels and choose those that at least contain real fruit or flavours. Most of the big foodstores sell their own diet ranges and you can choose your own from these. As a general rule, most small pots of low-fat yoghurt (such as the excellent Boots' Shapers range) tend to contain around 55Kcals, diet chocolate desserts (e.g. Sainsbury's) have around 60Kcals and diet fromage frais (e.g. Marks & Spencer's) around 50Kcals. Other desserts such as diet mousse and low-fat fool contain around 90Kcals per pot. Read the labels and check the calorie content before you buy as different brands can vary.

If you don't want to eat synthetic desserts, make your own versions using 4 tbsp low-fat, live, plain or naturally flavoured yoghurt sprinkled with 1tbsp chopped fruits. Very low-fat fromage frais is also a good, naturally healthy choice.

HANDY DESSERT OPTION

The following is a guide to the many kinds of low-calorie, low-fat desserts and yoghurts available from the shops.

Dessert	Kcals
Boots Shapers	
Very Low Fat Strawberry Yoghurt	53
Milk Chocolate Mousse	88
Strawberrry Yoghurt Mousse	55
St Michael	
Lite Very Low Fat Yoghurts:	
Strawberry and Raspberry	62
Mango	62
Strawberry and Vanilla	60
Peach and Starfruit	62
Nectarine and Orange	69
Rhubarb	63
Peach Melba	66
Pineapple	68
Vanilla	65
Raspberry Lite Fromage Frais	50
Apricot Lite Fromage Frais	51
Strawberry Lite Fromage Frais	51
Fruits of the Forest Fromage Frais	52
Lite Milk Chocolate Mousse	89
Lite Toffee Mousse	91
Sainsbury	
Lemon Diet Fromage Frais	45
Blackberry Diet Fromage Frais	45
Raspberry Diet Fromage Frais	45
Cherry Diet Bio Yoghurt	54
Strawberry Diet Bio Yoghurt	54
Peach and Passion-Fruit Diet Bio Yoghurt	54
Plum Diet Bio Yoghurt	54
Strawberry Low Fat Fool	89
Apricot Low Fat Fool	90
Diet Chocolate Mousse	59

Section 5

RECIPES

BREAKFAST

Fruit Compôte FC (P)

> *Serves 6*
> Per serving:
> Kcals   165
> Fat   0.8g
> Fibre   13g

This compôte is the ideal fast-food breakfast as it is prepared the day before, can be kept covered in the fridge for at least a week and is ready to serve immediately.

> *75g (3oz) dried apple rings*
> *75g (3oz) dried apricots*
> *75g (3oz) dried pears*
> *75g (3oz) prunes*
> *1/2 tsp allspice*
> *1/2 tsp cinnamon*
> *300ml (1/2 pint) water*
> *plain, low-fat bio yoghurt to serve*

Choose unsulphured dried fruit where possible (from health food shops), as this is preserved without sulphur dioxide. Soak the fruits and spices in the water overnight. Serve cold or slightly warmed, adding 1 tablespoonful of plain, low-fat bio yoghurt.

Summer Muesli

> *Serves 2*
> Per serving:
> Kcals   160
> Fat   5.7g
> Fibre   1.2g

This recipe is based on the original muesli invented by Dr Bircher-Benner for patients at his famous natural health spa in the Swiss Alps. To save time in the mornings, soak the oats overnight, leaving only the fruit and nuts to be added at breakfast. This is my favourite way to start the day.

    4 tbsp rolled porridge oats
    2 tbsp plain, low-fat bio yoghurt
    6 tsp water
    1 tsp grated lemon peel
    50g (2oz) freshly grated apple or 50g (2oz) seasonal summer fruits,
    such as strawberries
    1 tbsp chopped hazlenuts or almonds

Put the oats, yoghurt, water and lemon peel into a large bowl and stir until creamy. Leave in the fridge overnight if preferred. Add the fresh fruit and serve sprinkled with chopped hazelnuts or almonds.

Wake-up shake FC (N)

    Serves 1
    Per serving:
    Kcals   260
    Fat   16g
    Fibre   4.8g

This wake-up shake will boost your vitamin levels and give you extra energy at the start of the day. It tastes best chilled. Note that it is higher in calories than the other Bikini Diet breakfast options.

    1 level tbsp sunflower seeds
    1 level tbsp sesame seeds
    2 apples, peeled and cored
    1 teaspoon crude blackstrap molasses

Finely grind the seeds in a coffee mill or food processor. Liquidise the apples in the food processor and blend with the ground seeds and molasses. Serve immediately while still frothy. You will find the molasses in a health food shop, or you could use black treacle, although this is not as nutritious.

LUNCH

Asparagus and Parmesan Salad FC (P)

    Serves 6
    Per serving:
    Kcals   180
    Fat   16.2 g
    Fibre   0.75 g

This deluxe salad makes a delicious light lunch or a starter dish for a supper party. Some delicatessens sell dandelion leaves in the summer. Alternatively, you can either grow your own (avoid any use of weed killer!) or substitute salad rocket leaves.

> 225g (8oz) asparagus
> 1 handful fresh young dandelion leaves
> 2 heads chicory or small red radicchio lettuce
> 1 handful baby spinach leaves or rocket
> 100g (4oz) freshly grated Parmesan

Dressing:
> juice of 2 lemons
> 4 tbsp (60ml) sunflower oil
> salt and freshly ground black pepper

Blanch the asparagus in lightly salted, boiling water (3–6 mins), drain and allow to cool. Meanwhile, wash and thoroughly dry the salad leaves.

Make the salad dressing by mixing together the juice of the lemons and the sunflower oil and season to taste.

To combine the ingredients, place the salad leaves on the six plates and arrange the asparagus on top. Then pour over the dressing and sprinkle the shavings of Parmesan on top.

Avocado and Alfalfa Sandwich FC (C)

Serves 1

Kcals	220
Fat	10.9g
Fibre	3.7g

A luxurious sandwich recipe which will fill you up with goodness.

> 1/2 an avocado
> 1/2 a spring onion, finely chopped
> dash lemon juice
> freshly ground black pepper
> 2 thin slices wholemeal bread
> large handful alfalfa sprouts

Mash the avocado with the spring onion, lemon juice and black pepper and spread on a slice of bread. Sprinkle with alfalfa sprouts and top with the second slice of wholemeal bread.

Chicken Stuffed with Spinach and Cheese FC (P)

Serves 4
Per serving:

Kcals	305
Fat	13.5g
Fibre	2.2g

> 225g (8oz) spinach
> 1–2 cloves garlic, crushed
> 100g (4oz) low-fat cottage cheese
> 1/2 tsp nutmeg

salt and pepper to season
4 boneless, skinless chicken breasts

Pre-heat the oven to 200°C/400°F/gas mark 6. Wash the spinach, remove any tough stalks and place in a medium-sized saucepan, together with the garlic. Cover with the lid and cook over a medium to low heat for 3–4 minutes. The spinach will wilt and soften just in the water that clings to the leaves. Drain away any excess liquid and allow to cool a little. Chop the spinach and mix with the cottage cheese, nutmeg and seasoning. Cut a horizontal slice three-quarters of the way through the chicken to form a 'pocket', stuff in the spinach filling. Place in a non-stick roasting tin, pour over a cup of water or stock and cover with tin foil. Cook in the oven for 20–30 minutes until juices run clear when the thickest part of the fillet is pierced.

Veggie variation: Use the spinach filling to stuff aubergines, peppers or large field mushrooms, adding a little cooked rice and a sprinkling of pine nuts or almonds. **FC (C)**

Chilled Melon with Parma Ham and Strawberry Salsa FC (P)

Serves 4
Per serving:

Kcal	190
Fat	10.2g
Fibre	3.4g

Everyone knows that strawberries are sweet, but did you realise that this delicious fruit can be turned to savoury use? For this recipe I have combined sweet strawberries with black pepper, orange and ginger to make a savoury salsa.Try it with slices of cold fragrant melon draped with slices of Parma ham for an exotic summer lunch. It's also good with leftover cold chicken.

1 large ripe melon – cantaloupe, galia, or charentais, chilled
175g (6oz) Parma, Serrano ham or similar
Strawberry salsa:
225g (8oz) ripe strawberries
1 tsp caster sugar
2 tbsp groundnut (peanut) or soya oil
1/2 tsp finely grated orange zest
1 tbsp orange juice
1/2 tsp finely grated fresh root ginger
salt and freshly ground black pepper to season

Halve the melon and take out the seeds with a spoon. Cut the rind away with a paring knife, then slice the melon thickly. Chill until ready to serve. To make the salsa, hull the strawberries, and cut them into large dice shapes. Place them in a mixing bowl with the sugar and crush lightly to release the juices. Add the oil, orange zest, juice and ginger. Season with salt and a generous twist of black pepper. Arrange the melon on a serving plate, drape the ham over the top and let your guests help themselves to the salsa.

Quick tip: Strawberry salsa is delicious served with grilled white fish, chicken and pork. It is also good served as a relish with cold meats, so keep a pot handy in the fridge for an instant summer meal.

Cold Summer Omelette FC (P)

Serves 1 – makes 1 omelette

Kcals   244
Fat   23.7g
Fibre   0.6g

1 small tomato
1 large egg
salt and freshly ground black pepper
15g (¹/₂ oz) butter
chopped parsley

Skin the tomato, remove the seeds, chop and season. Break the egg into a bowl, add a little salt and pepper and whisk. Heat a 15cm (6") omelette pan, add the butter and when melted, add the egg. Add the tomato and fold into the omelette. When the egg is cooked, fold it in three using a palette knife and transfer to a plate. Allow to cool and serve with some salad and chopped parsley.

Endive and Apple Salad FC (N)

Serves 6

Per serving:
Kcals   173
Fat   15.2g
Fibre   2.0g

This unusual salad really is a treat for the taste-buds. The delicately bitter flavour of the endives and walnuts works very well with the sweetness of the honey and apples.

50g (2oz) walnut pieces
6 endives, bottoms trimmed
2 apples, cored and diced
salt and freshly ground pepper
50g (2oz) sunflower seeds

Dressing:
1 tsp (5ml) honey
1 tsp (5ml) Dijon mustard
1 tbsp (15ml) cider vinegar
2 tbsp (30ml) extra-virgin olive oil

To prepare the walnuts, preheat the oven to 300F/150°C/gas mark 2. Place the walnuts pieces on a baking sheet and toast in the oven for 4 minutes. Remove and allow to cool. Meanwhile, remove the large outer leaves of the endives and put them to one side before slicing the remaining leaves.

To make the dressing, whisk together the honey, mustard, cider vinegar and olive oil in a salad bowl and season to taste. Add the walnuts, sliced apples and endives to the bowl and toss in the dressing. The salad can now be arranged on a platter or serving dish. First position the large outer leaves of the endives around the edge of the dish, then spoon the salad mixture into the centre and sprinkle with sunflower seeds.

Great Green Salad FC (N)

Serves 4
Per serving:

Kcals	36
Fat	0.9 g
Fibre	2.9 g

This salad is bursting with vitamins and minerals and the rocket, spring onions and watercress give it a tasty, spicy flavour.

1 bunch watercress
1 cos or frisée lettuce
50g (2oz) salad rocket
1/2 medium-sized cauliflower
1 bunch spring onions, thinly sliced
100g (4oz) bean sprouts
100g (4oz) mushrooms, sliced
Dressing (see pages 128–9)

Wash and prepare all the vegetables, separate the watercress into sprigs and chop the stalks finely. Tear the lettuce and rocket into small pieces and break the cauliflower into very small florets.

Then simply toss the salad in 4 tsp (20 ml) of a *Bikini Diet* dressing.

Greek Spring Salad FC (P)

Serves 4
Per serving:

Kcals	190
Fat	9.2g
Fibre	5.7g

450g (16oz) raw spinach, baby leaves if possible
175g (6oz) low-fat cottage cheese
50g (2oz) currants
50g (2oz) black olives, pitted
50g (2oz) radishes, thinly sliced
4 spring onions, sliced lengthways
Dressing:
1 tbsp sunflower oil
1 tbsp lemon juice

1 tbsp sesame seeds
1 clove garlic, crushed
1 tsp fresh oregano, chopped
salt and black pepper to season

Rinse and dry the spinach. Tear the larger leaves into bite-sized pieces, discarding any stringy stems. Place in a large salad bowl, add the cheese, currants, black olives and radishes. Mix the dressing ingredients together and pour over the salad. Toss well and garnish with the spring onions.

Green Bean and Bacon Salad FC (P)

Serves 4
Per serving:

Kcals	150
Fat	6.4g
Fibre	4.6g

This colourful salad makes a tasty light lunch or a good accompaniment to a baked jacket potato.

450g (16oz) green beans, trimmed and sliced into 5.5cm (2") lengths
4 rashers lean bacon, rind removed
1 red pepper, de-seeded and roughly chopped
1 small onion, finely chopped

Dressing

150ml (16oz) natural low-fat yoghurt
1 tbsp olive oil
1 tbsp lemon juice
1 tsp mustard
2 tbsp chopped chives
1 clove garlic, crushed
freshly ground black pepper

Steam or microwave the beans in a small amount of water until tender, but still crisp. Grill the bacon and cut into bite-sized pieces. Mix the beans, bacon, chopped raw onion and red pepper together. Stir all the dressing ingredients together and whisk. Pour the dressing over the salad and stir well.

Halibut Salad with Lemon and Herb Dressing FC (P)

Serves 4
Per serving:

Kcals	216
Fat	4g
Fibre	0.8g

Halibut is the tastiest fish to use in this deluxe recipe, but it also works well with cod or hoki (an inexpensive fish from New Zealand).

    1 firm lettuce
    450g (1lb) cooked halibut steaks
    1 bunch radishes
Dressing:
    pinch of salt, freshly ground pepper
    1 tsp dill, oregano or basil, finely chopped
    grated rind and juice of 1/2 lemon
    1tsp olive oil
    75ml (3fl oz) low-fat fromage frais

Simply separate the washed lettuce leaves on to four plates and arrange the halibut steaks and radishes on top. Then to make the herb dressing, whisk the salt, pepper, herbs and lemon rind in the lemon juice with a fork until the salt has dissolved. Then add the oil, whisk the mixture until the oil is combined and finally stir in the fromage frais until you have a creamy sauce – take care not to over stir or it will thicken too much. Pour the dressing over the salad and serve.

Herbed Mushrooms FC (N)

    Serves 4–6

Kcals	220
Fat	22.2g
Fibre:	1.8g

These mushrooms are delicious served alone as a starter or as a salad ingredient. They can also be drained and served warm as a vegetable side dish.

    450g (1lb) mushrooms
    250ml (8fl oz) red wine vinegar
    100g (4oz) onions, finely chopped
    1 tsp mixed spice, pickling spice or allspice
    4 cloves
    100g (4oz) red pepper, de-seeded and sliced
    120ml (4fl oz) sunflower oil
    salt and freshly ground black pepper

Lightly brush the mushrooms with a damp cloth to remove any earth. Blanch by plunging briefly into boiling water for 20 seconds. Drain and allow to cool. Meanwhile, bring the vinegar to the boil in a non-aluminium pan. Add the chopped onions and seasonings. Cook for 2–3 minutes before adding the sliced red pepper, sunflower oil and salt and pepper. Cool the mixture, add the mushrooms and leave to marinade for 2–3 hours. Drain the oil and juices before serving. The mushrooms can be stored in a screw-top jar in the refrigerator for at least a fortnight.

Low-Calorie Tricolore FC (N)

Serves 2
Per serving:
Kcals   148
Fat   8.9g
Fibre   2.9g

This deliciously light salad is a variation of the classic Italian mozzarella and tomato salad, but is far lower in fat.

450g (1lb) tomatoes
100g (4oz) low-fat cottage cheese
20 fresh basil leaves
1 tbsp extra virgin olive oil
salt and freshly ground black pepper

If you prefer your tomatoes skinless, the best method of skinning is to make a couple of small slits in the skins, place in a bowl and pour boiling water over them. Leave them for exactly 1 minute, drain and the skin should come away easily. Slice the tomatoes thinly.

On a serving dish, arrange the tomato slices, leaving a space for a small scoop of cottage cheese between each slice. Then scatter the basil leaves on top. Before serving, add a couple of drops of olive oil and sprinkle with plenty of salt and pepper. Serve with a couple of rice cakes or a wholemeal pitta bread. **(C)**

Low-fat Chicken Liver Pâté FC (P)

Serves 4
Per serving:
Kcals   145
Fat   7.3g
Fibre   0.3g

1 onion, chopped
1 clove garlic, crushed
1 tbsp olive oil
200g (7oz) chicken livers
1/2 glass red wine or vegetable stock
2 tbsp wholegrain mustard

Sauté the onion and garlic in olive oil, add the chicken livers. Cook until browned before adding the red wine or vegetable stock. Season with salt, pepper and wholegrain mustard. Cook for 10–15 minutes. Chop finely or purée in a food processor, cool and serve with toast, crackers and salad or sticks of carrot and celery.

Low-fat Hummous

Serves 4
Per serving:
Kcals   182
Fat   6.6g
Fibre   4.7g

Hummous is a great Greek pâté of chickpeas, olive oil, garlic and lemon. You can boil your own chickpeas but it's quicker to use tinned ones.

420g (15oz) can chickpeas, drained
1–2 cloves garlic, crushed
2 tbsp lemon juice
1 tbsp olive oil
pinch cayenne pepper
150ml (5floz) low-fat live yoghurt

Place all the ingredients in a food processor and blend until smooth, taste and add a little more seasoning or lemon juice if needed. Serve with a selection of raw vegetables, 'crudités'. Choose from carrots, celery, cucumber, peppers, broccoli, cauliflower, mushrooms, courgette etc. The more the merrier. There are so few calories in the vegetables you can eat as much you like.

Quick tip: Freeze portions in empty yoghurt pots ready for a quick lunch.

Mackerel Fillets FC (P)

Serves 4
Per serving:
Kcals   409
Fat   33.9g
Fibre   1.4g
2 large mackerel, filleted
2 tbsp Parmesan cheese, grated
2 cloves garlic, crushed
juice and rind of 1 large lemon
2–3 tbsp chopped fresh parsley

Rinse the mackerel fillets and place skin side down in a large, greased ovenproof dish. In a bowl, mix together the Parmesan cheese, garlic, the juice and rind of the lemon and the parsley. Spread the paste over the fillets and cook in the oven or microwave. Serve with a selection of summer vegetables.

No-Cook Rissoles FC (C)

Serves 4 – makes 8 small rissoles
Kcals   449
Fat   34.2g
Fibre: 5.2g

Serve these rissoles with one delicious neutral salad meal.

175g (6oz) mixed nuts (eg hazelnuts and almonds), ground
100g (4oz) wholewheat breadcrumbs
1 dessertspoon finely chopped onion
1 tbsp chopped parsley
1 tsp low-salt yeast extract blended with 1 tsp water
1 dessertspoon poppy or sesame seeds

Reserve about one-quarter of the nuts and breadcrumbs for coating, and mix all the remaining ingredients together. Form into small rissoles. Mix together the reserved nuts and breadcrumbs and use to coat the rissoles.

Pitta Bread Salad FC (C)

Serves 4
Per serving:

Kcals	510
Fat	37.2g
Fibre	6.3g

This colourful salad is loaded with nutrients and the fresh herbs and mustard dressing make it really tasty. The pitta bread pieces are a good source of carbohydrates and will give you the slow release energy you need to keep hunger pangs at bay for hours.

2 small baby courgettes, finely chopped
1 small lettuce, roughly chopped
175g (6oz) cherry tomatoes
1 cucumber, chopped into bite-size chunks
6 tbsp parsley, chopped
2 tbsp chopped mint
4 spring onions, thinly sliced
1 small red onion, finely diced
2 wholemeal pitta breads

Dressing:
150ml (5fl oz) sunflower or hazelnut oil
zest of 1 lemon
4 tbsp fresh lemon juice
1 tsp French mustard
salt and freshly ground black pepper to season

Mix the chopped herbs and vegetables together in a large salad bowl. In a separate bowl or jug, whisk together all the ingredients for the dressing and season well. Spoon the dressing over the salad and toss thoroughly.

Grill the pitta bread until crisp, cut into small pieces and add to the salad. Toss the salad once more, season to taste and serve immediately to prevent the pitta bread turning soggy.

Potato, Bean and Pepperoni Salad

Serves 4
Per serving:
Kcals   185
Fat   1.9g
Fibre   8.6g
450g (1lb) small new potatoes
225g (8oz) shelled broad beans
225g (8oz) green beans, sliced
3 tbsp low-fat live yoghurt
few drops Tabasco sauce
1 small red onion, thinly sliced
50g (2oz) pepperoni, thinly sliced
3 tbsp flat parsley leaves, chopped
225g (8oz) green salad leaves, e.g. lettuce, watercress, rocket

Cook the potatoes in just enough water to cover them, for four minutes. Add the broad beans and green beans and continue cooking, covered, for a further 3 minutes. Drain and tip into a bowl. Add the yoghurt and Tabasco sauce, mix well and leave to cool. Add the red onion, pepperoni and parsley and stir lightly. Serve on a bed of green salad leaves.

Ratatouille and Pasta Salad FC (C)

Serves 4
Per serving:
Kcals   260
Fat   1.0g
Fibre   7.5g
175g (6oz) wholemeal pasta shapes
1 tbsp olive oil
1–2 tbsp balsamic vinegar or lemon juice
150g (5oz) ratatouille (see recipe on page 113)

This recipe is a good way to use up leftover pasta and/or ratatouille. Cook the pasta shapes (or use leftover pasta), drain and rinse in cold water. Toss in the olive oil and balsamic vinegar. Add the ratatouille (tinned is fine), mix and serve.

Red Pepper with Tagliatelle and Vegetables FC (C)

Serves 4
Per serving:
Kcals   186
Fat   5.5g
Fibre   5.5g
1 onion, chopped
2 cloves garlic, sliced

1 large red pepper, de-seeded and sliced
1–2 tbsp olive oil
4 ripe tomatoes, skinned and chopped
few basil leaves
275g (10oz) tagliatelle or linguini
450g (1lb) vegetables (courgettes, carrots, celery, spring onions)
25g (1oz) black olives, halved

Sauté the chopped onion, garlic and red pepper in the oil until softened but not browned. Add the tomatoes, half the basil and 2–3 tablespoons of water and cook for 4–5 minutes. Blend the sauce to a smooth purée. Meanwhile, cook the pasta in a large pan of boiling water or vegetable stock, for extra flavour. Cut the vegetables into very fine 'tagliatelle' strips and add to the pasta for the last two minutes of cooking time, so they cook but retain a little crunch. Drain the pasta and vegetables and serve with the sauce, garnish with the black olives and basil leaves.

Roast Vegetable Kebabs with Nutty Rice FC (C)

Serves 4
Per serving:

Kcals	239
Fat	10.8g
Fibre	5.4g

1 fennel bulb
1 onion
1 yellow pepper
1 red pepper
1 large courgette
1 medium aubergine
100g (4oz) small mushrooms
8 tiny tomatoes
1 tbsp olive oil
225g (8oz) preferably organic brown rice
vegetable stock
1 tbsp cashew nut pieces
1 tbsp sesame seeds
1 tbsp sunflower seeds
2 tbsp mixed dried herbs

Prepare the fennel, courgette, aubergine, peppers, mushrooms, tomatoes and onion and cut into pieces, threading alternatively on to kebab skewers. Brush with 1 tbsp olive oil and sprinkle with the dried mixed herbs. Grill or barbecue until softened and browned at the edges. Meanwhile cook the rice in vegetable stock, toast the sunflower seeds, sesame seeds and cashew nuts in a pan under the grill and toss into the rice. Serve the rice with the cooked kebabs.

Smoked Mackerel, Pasta and Apple Salad

Serves 4
Per serving:
Kcals   371
Fat   20.5g
Fibre   2.7g

This mighty salad is rich in protein and carbohydrate and is really filling, though low in calories.

450 g (1lb) wholemeal pasta shapes
6 tbsp low-fat, plain yoghurt
2–3 tbsp lemon juice
2 eating apples, cored and diced
6 spring onions, trimmed and sliced
1–2 tsp dill seeds
225 g (8oz) smoked mackerel fillets (cooked)
freshly ground black pepper
chopped fresh parsley to garnish

Cook the pasta in a large pan of salted water. Meanwhile, whisk together the yoghurt and lemon juice in a large mixing bowl, and add the apple, spring onions and dill seeds. Remove the skin from the smoked mackerel fillets, cut into strips and set aside. Drain the cooked pasta and add to the mixing bowl, folding together all the ingredients with a large wooden spoon. Season with freshly ground black pepper. Allow to cool and then add the smoked mackerel strips, mixing gently so that the flakes do not break up. Serve immediately garnished with fresh parsley.

Spanish Omelette

Serves 4
Per serving:
Kcals   205
Fat   9.0g
Fibre   2.0g

1 medium onion, sliced
1 clove garlic, crushed
450g (1lb) diced, cooked new potatoes
4 beaten eggs
1 tbsp olive oil
seasoning

Sauté the sliced onion and crushed clove of garlic in the oil, then add the potatoes. When browned, pour over the eggs and add seasoning according to taste. Cook slowly until just firm before browning under the grill. A delicious snack which can be served hot or cold.

Spinach and Prosciutto Salad FC (P)

Serves 4
Per serving:
Kcals   109
Fat   5.9g
Fibre   3.4g
100g (4oz) prosciutto ham or similar
350g (12oz) baby spinach leaves
50g (2oz) Emmental cheese or similar
3 tbsp low-calorie vinaigrette

Cut the ham into strips and add to the baby spinach leaves together with the finely diced cheese. Toss in the low-calorie dressing and serve.

Stuffed Mediterranean Tomatoes FC (P)

Serves 4
Per serving:
Kcals   170
Fat   1.7g
Fibre   4.6g
4 large beefsteak tomatoes
320g (11oz) can of sweetcorn, drained
200g (7oz) can of tuna in brine, drained
2 tbsp low-calorie mayonnaise

Slice the top off the tomatoes and scoop out the seeds. Mix together the sweetcorn with the tuna. Add the mayonnaise and pile into the tomatoes.

Stuffed Tomato Salad FC (N)

Serves 2
Per serving:
Kcals   29
Fat   0.6g
Fibre   3.5g
1 green pepper, finely chopped
1 stick celery, finely chopped
1/4 medium-sized onion, finely chopped
2 tbsp freshly chopped parsley
4 large firm, ripe tomatoes
few drops olive oil and vinegar dressing
slices of lemon to garnish

Mix the diced pepper, celery, onion and parsley together in a bowl with a few drops of olive oil and vinegar dressing. Then remove the tops of the tomatoes, scoop out the seeds and central flesh and add this to the other ingredients.

The shell of the tomatoes are left behind and can now be stuffed with the vegetable mixture. Garnish with a slice of lemon, and serve with a couple of crispbreads or rice cakes. **FC (C)**

Sunshine Salad FC (N)

Serves 6
Per serving:
Kcals   240
Fat   22.8g
Fibre   4.3g

This salad makes an attractive starter or light lunch dish and it's really healthy! You can adapt the recipe according to the salad leaves and fresh herbs available.

Dressing:
   100ml (3¹/2fl oz) olive oil or sunflower oil
   25ml (1fl oz) fresh lemon or lime juice
   2 tsp mustard
   freshly ground black pepper

Salad:
   4 large carrots, scrubbed and grated
   225g (8oz) mixed salad leaves, such as spinach, radicchio, frisée, oakleaf and batavia lettuces, endive and corn salad or lamb's lettuce
   50g (2oz) mixed herb leaves, such as chervil, basil and rocket
   50g (2oz) sun-dried tomatoes, finely chopped
   50g (2oz) hazelnuts, almonds or pecans, finely chopped

Mix together the dressing ingredients. Pour half the dressing over the grated carrots. Put the carrots in the centre of a large, flat serving platter. Arrange the mixed salad and herb leaves round the outside. Sprinkle with the chopped, sun-dried tomatoes and nuts. Pour on the remaining salad dressing and serve immediately.

Tabbouleh FC (C)

Serves 6
Per serving:
Kcals   188
Fat   6.5g
Fibre   3.4g

This is a popular Middle Eastern salad dish which can be prepared in advance and keeps well in a covered container in the fridge.

   175g (6oz) bulgar wheat (cracked wheat)
   4 spring onions, trimmed and finely chopped
   1 medium-sized cucumber, finely chopped
   4 tbsp finely chopped parsley
   1–2 tbsp freshly chopped mint
   1–2 tbsp freshly chopped basil

freshly squeezed juice of 1 lemon
2 tbsp olive or hazelnut oil for extra flavour
6 slivers red pepper or pimento to garnish

Rinse the bulgar wheat before soaking it in cold water for at least an hour. Drain well. Add the finely chopped spring onions, cucumber and herbs to the lemon juice and oil and mix together well. Pour the mixture over the bulgar wheat and stir thoroughly. Serve garnished with slivers of red pepper or pimento.

Tahini and Cucumber Sandwich FC (C)

Serves 1

Kcals	165
Fat	5.5g
Fibre	1.0g

Tahini spread is made from crushed sesame seeds. It is very high in calcium and is available from good supermarkets and health-food shops. It is also high in fat, so use sparingly.

$1/2$ tbsp of tahini spread
1 tsp chopped parsley
6 cucumber slices
2 thin slices wholemeal bread

Spread the tahini on to one of the slices of wholemeal bread. Sprinkle with the chopped parsley and place the cucumber and the other slice of bread on top. Serve with cherry tomatoes, radishes and spring onions.

Tangy Tuna Salad

Serves 4–6
Per serving:

Kcals	260
Fat	6.5g
Fibre	12.2g

Tuna fish and beans are a great source of protein. This simple salad is tasty and filling, and gives you the energy you need without being high in calories.

2 x 200g (7oz) cans tuna in brine, drained
2 x 400g (14oz) cans cannellini or kidney beans
3 spring onions, thinly sliced
1 red pepper, roughly diced
2 tbsp extra virgin olive oil
2 tbsp fresh lemon juice
1 tbsp chopped fresh parsley
salt and freshly ground black pepper

Separate the tuna into large flakes and place in a large salad bowl or serving dish. Strain and rinse the beans under cold water, drain, and add to the tuna. Then sprinkle the spring onions and chopped red pepper over the beans.

For a deliciously simple dressing, just mix the oil with the lemon juice, add the parsley, season with salt and pepper and mix thoroughly before pouring over the salad. Toss well before serving.

Tomato and Feta Cheese Salad FC (P)

Serves 4
Per serving:
Kcals   235
Fat   18.3g
Fibre   3.2g

When buying feta cheese look for Greek and Turkish brands as European feta cheese can be over-salted. Low-fat feta is also available from some supermarkets.

1kg (2lb) tomatoes
200g (7oz) feta cheese
2 tbsp olive oil
1 small bunch fresh basil
8 black olives (optional)

Slice the tomatoes and arrange on a serving plate. Scatter with olive oil, crumble on the feta cheese and add the olives. Just before you are ready to serve, tear the basil leaves and toss them over the cheese. Tearing basil leaves releases a good flavour and they blacken less quickly.

Tomato and Vegetable Soup FC (N)

Serves 4
Per serving:
Kcals   23
Fat   0.6g
Fibre   1.8g

100g (4oz) celery, chopped, with its leaves
100g (4oz) carrot, grated
50g (2oz) raw spinach, finely grated
1ltr (1³/₄pts) water
125ml (4fl oz) tomato juice
1tsp honey
1/2 tsp cayenne pepper
1 tbsp chopped chives

Boil the water in a pan and add the chopped vegetables. Cover, turn down the heat and simmer for 20–30 minutes. Add the tomato juice, honey and cayenne pepper. Pour into a blender and liquidise until smooth. Serve with a sprinkling of chopped chives.

Tomato, Avocado and Mozzarella Salad FC (P)

Serves 4
Per serving:
Kcals   140
Fat   11.8g
Fibre   3.3g
4 large beefsteak tomatoes
1 medium avocado
100g (4oz) reduced-fat mozzarella cheese
fresh basil leaves to garnish
2 tbsp low-calorie vinaigrette or yoghurt and chive dressing
  (see recipe page 129)

Slice the tomatoes, avocado and mozzarella cheese. Arrange in alternating slices on a plate. Pour over 2 tbsp of low-fat dressing and serve.

Tropical Fish Salad with a Hot Mango Dressing FC (P)

Serves 4
Per serving:
Kcals   395
Fat   10.4g
Fibre   3.4g

If you were on a dream holiday somewhere hot and tropical, the chances are you would eat nothing but fresh fish, salad and fruit. The chances of taking such a holiday may be slim, but here is an opportunity to indulge in an exotic feast of your own. A fishmonger will prepare the fish to make life easier.

4 black bream, red fish or mullet, scaled and gutted, each weighing about
  275g (10oz)
2 tbsp olive oil
salt and freshly ground black pepper to season
Mango dressing:
1 large ripe mango
1cm (1/2") fresh root ginger, peeled and chopped
1/2 tsp chilli paste
2 tbsp lemon or lime juice
3 tbsp freshly chopped coriander leaf
1 batavian, endive or escarole lettuce
75g (3oz) lamb's lettuce or corn salad
12 cherry tomatoes, halved

Pre-heat a moderate grill or light a barbecue and let the embers settle to a steady glow. Slash the fish deeply on both sides, brush lightly with oil, season well and set aside. To make the mango dressing, remove the top and bottom from the flat oval of the mango, stand on one cut end and pare away the thin skin. Remove the flesh from both sides of the flat fibrous stone. Slice one half of the mango flesh for use in the salad later, and put the remainder in a food processor with the ginger, lime, chilli and coriander. Process until smooth. Transfer to a serving dish and set aside. Put the fish on to grill or barbecue for 6–8 minutes turning once. Wash the salad leaves and dry, then distribute between four large plates. Place a fish on each and decorate with slices of mango and tomato.

Tuna-stuffed Pitta Pocket

Serves 1

Kcals   294
Fat   1.5g
Fibre   5.0g

50g (2oz) tuna
1 tbsp onion, finely chopped
2 tbsp alfalfa sprouts
2 tsp reduced-calorie mayonnaise or low-fat fromage frais
1 wholemeal pitta bread
2 lettuce leaves, shredded

Mix together the tuna, onion, alfalfa sprouts and mayonnaise. Slice the pitta bread in half to create two pockets. Line each pocket with shredded lettuce and stuff with the tuna fish mixture.

Turkish Boregs with a Minty Yoghurt Sauce

Serves 4
Per serving:

Kcals   744
Fat   45g
Fibre   3.2g

The boreg is the Eastern Mediterranean equivalent to our Cornish pasty. In Turkey they are filled with couscous and a host of seasonal flavours. The pastry contains little saturated fat and is easy to make and handle. Because boregs are so quick to put together, they are ideal for last-minute summer picnics or packed lunches. Couscous is available in all good supermarkets and health-food stores. You can reduce the fat content by using low-fat feta cheese.

400g (14oz) self-raising flour
1tsp salt
150ml (5fl oz) olive oil
150ml (5 fl oz) low-fat yoghurt
1 egg
Filling:
175g (6oz) couscous
350ml (12fl oz) boiling water
1 egg
1tsp ground cinnamon

    1tsp ground coriander
    1 tsp celery salt or a pinch of ordinary salt
    $1/4$ tsp cayenne pepper
    1 small bunch parsley, chopped
    100g (4oz) feta cheese, crumbled
    5 tbsp olive oil
    1 beaten egg to glaze
Minty yoghurt sauce:
    150ml (5fl oz) low-fat yoghurt
    12 large mint leaves, chopped
    $1/2$ tsp caster sugar

Pre-heat the oven to 200°C/400°F/gas mark 6. To make the filling, place the couscous in a large bowl, cover with boiling water and leave for 10 minutes until the water is absorbed. In the meantime hard-boil the egg for 12 minutes, cool under running water, shell and roughly chop. Add to the couscous with the remaining ingredients and fold together with a large spoon. To make the pastry, sieve the flour and salt into a hand-mixing bowl. Measure the oil and yoghurt into a measuring jug, add the egg and beat together. Add the contents of the jug to the flour and stir to make a scone-like pastry. Turn the pastry onto a floured work surface and divide into four. Roll each into a 15cm (6") round and divide the couscous filling between them. Turn over and press lightly with the fingers of one hand. Brush the boregs with the beaten egg (a good pinch of salt beaten into the egg will improve the glaze) and bake in the pre-heated oven for 20 minutes. Allow to cool to room temperature and serve with minted yoghurt sauce made by combining the freshly chopped mint, yoghurt and sugar.

Warm Goat's Cheese Salad FC (P)

    Serves 4
    Per serving:

Kcals	214
Fat	19g
Fibre	1.0g

    175g (6oz) goat's cheese
    1 tbsp olive oil
    16 mixed salad leaves
    50g (2oz) sunflower seeds
    2 tbsp fine French dressing (see recipe page 128)

Pre-heat the grill or the oven to 180°C/350°F/gas mark 4 .

    Slice the goat's cheese into four thick slices. Brush a baking tray with the olive oil and place the cheese slices on it. Heat in the oven or under a medium grill until melted and lightly brown. Meanwhile, toss the salad leaves in the dressing and arrange on four small plates. Place one slice of goat's cheese in the centre. Sprinkle with sunflower seeds and serve immediately, while still warm.

DINNER
VEGETARIAN

Basmati Vegetable Pilaf FC (C)

Serves 4
Per serving:
Kcals   233
Fat   11.4g
Fibre   6.9g

Fresh vegetables are full of the vitality vitamins we need to stay fit and healthy. This delicious dish is loaded with the veggies we know we should eat more of!

3 tbsp olive oil
1 medium onion, chopped
1 tsp ground coriander
$^1/_2$ tsp ground cinnamon
1 pinch ground allspice
275g (10oz) basmati rice
600ml (1 pint) vegetable stock
750g (1lb 8oz) young vegetables, to include: baby sweetcorn, carrots, green beans, broccoli, sugar snap peas (or mange-tout) and courgettes
dash of soy sauce

To prepare the vegetables, peel, trim and halve the carrots, top and tail and halve the beans, cut the broccoli into florets, top and tail the sugar snap peas, trim and slice the courgettes. Heat the oil in a large wok or saucepan, add the onion and soften without browning. Add the coriander, cinnamon and allspice, then stir in the rice until evenly coated. Pour in the vegetable stock, stir briefly and simmer for 10 minutes. Add the vegetables and cook for a further 5 minutes. Switch off the heat, cover and leave to finish cooking in its heat. If you don't have an enormous wok lid, cover the surface of the rice with a large circle of greaseproof paper lightly brushed with olive oil. Serve the pilaf in a generous bowl with a few shakes of soy sauce. Jasmine tea is a favourite of mine to accompany this delicious pilaf (and doesn't contain any calories!)

Buckwheat Bonanza FC (C)

Serves 2
Per serving:
Kcals   250
Fat   9.5g
Fibre   2.2g

This buckwheat feast works well with the stronger flavours of wild mushrooms such as shiitake or oyster varieties.

50g (2oz) roasted buckwheat (kasha)
50g (2oz) buckwheat
450ml (3/4 pint) water
100g (4oz) artichoke hearts
1 tbsp cold-pressed olive oil
100g (4oz) button or wild mushrooms, roughly chopped
4 spring onions, chopped
1 tsp dried sage and parsley
2 tsp chopped fresh sage and parsley
1 tsp tamari sauce
freshly ground black pepper
25g (1oz) pecan nuts (optional)

Rinse the buckwheat in a sieve under a running tap. Bring the water to the boil, add the buckwheat, cover and simmer for 15 minutes or until soft.

Meanwhile, if using fresh artichokes, trim and cook them in mineral water or in a steamer. When soft, remove the leaves and trim away the toughened fibres to reveal the soft hearts. If using tinned artichoke hearts these will be pre-cooked. Roughly chop the artichokes. In a large frying-pan heat the oil and gently soften the mushrooms and spring onions. Drain and add the buckwheat, chopped artichokes and herbs and stir well. Add the tamari sauce, and freshly ground black pepper to season. Serve sprinkled with pecan nuts, if using.

Cabbage Parcels FC (C)

Serves 6
Per serving:

Kcals	190
Fat	4.5g
Fibre	4.7g

100g (4oz) millet
450ml (15fl oz) vegetable stock
1 Savoy cabbage
8 stems of fresh coriander
1 tbsp cold-pressed olive oil
2 red onions, peeled and chopped
4 spring onions, sliced into rings
2 cloves garlic, peeled and crushed
3 carrots, chopped
2 leeks, chopped
4 tomatoes, chopped
100g (4oz) okra, chopped
juice of 1 lime
freshly ground black pepper
2 tbsp (30ml) water or stock

Pre-heat the oven to 180°C/350°F/gas mark 4.

Place the millet and stock in a saucepan, bring to the boil, cover and simmer for about twenty minutes or until the millet is soft.

Separate the cabbage into the whole leaves and blanch them in boiling water for 30 seconds. Set aside to drain on kitchen paper.

Slice the stems off the coriander. Chop the leaves and set on one side. Heat the oil and gently fry the onion, coriander stems and garlic until the onion is transparent. Add the chopped carrots and leeks and continue to cook for another minute. Add the tomatoes, okra, the chopped coriander leaves and stir in the cooked millet. Add the lime juice, and freshly ground black pepper.

Place a dessertspoonful of the millet mixture on a cabbage leaf and roll up, folding in the sides as you go. Repeat until all the cabbage leaves have been filled. Place in an ovenproof dish, spoon over 2 tablespoons of water or stock, cover and bake for 20 minutes.

Five Vegetable Terrine FC (P)

Serves 6–8
Per serving:

Kcals	120
Fat	6.2g
Fibre	3.5g

This multi-coloured terrine may be served hot or cold. For an attractive starter, slice and serve it in the centre of a plate of freshly squeezed tomato juice.

450g (1lb) carrots, diced
225g (8oz) celeriac, peeled and cubed
350g (12oz) fresh spinach
350g (12oz) broccoli, broken into florets
225g (8oz) leeks, white part only, sliced
freshly ground black pepper
6 free-range eggs, size 3
juice of 1 orange

Pre-heat the oven to 200°C/400°F/gas mark 6.

Cook the carrots and celeriac in boiling water in separate saucepans until tender. Cook the spinach in a little water for about 5–6 minutes. Blanch the broccoli and leeks in boiling water, separately, for 1–2 minutes. Drain all the vegetables well.

In a food processor, blend the leek and celeriac with a pinch of black pepper and two eggs until puréed to a coarse texture. Repeat, using the broccoli, spinach and two more of the eggs. Finally, repeat the process with the carrot, adding the orange juice and two remaining eggs.

Line a 1kg (2lb) loaf tin with lightly oiled baking parchment paper. Spread the green spinach and broccoli mixture over the bottom and follow with a cream-coloured layer of leek and celeriac. Finally, top with a layer of carrot and orange purée. Place the loaf tin inside a large roasting tin filled with about 1cm (½") of hot water. Bake for about 1 hour or until set. Turn out on a serving dish, allow to cool slightly then peel off the baking parchment before slicing the terrine.

Risotto-Stuffed Aubergines with a Spicy Tomato Sauce FC (C)

Serves 4
Per serving:

Kcals	379
Fat	28.3g
Fibre	3.6g

4 small, fat aubergines (approx. 15cm (6") long)
5 tbsp olive oil
1 clove garlic, crushed
2cm (1") fresh root ginger, peeled and chopped
175ml (6oz) short-grain rice (arborio or carnaroli)
600ml (1pint) vegetable stock
1 tbsp white wine vinegar

Sauce:
500ml (17fl oz) carton of puréed tomato (passata)
1 tsp ground coriander
1 tsp ground cumin
½ tsp fresh thyme
¼ tsp cayenne pepper

Topping:
25g (1oz) pine nuts
25g (1oz) Parmesan cheese, grated
3 tbsp roughly chopped parsley
4 sprigs basil leaves to garnish

Pre-heat the oven to 190°C/375°F/gas mark 5.

Cut the aubergines in half length-ways through the stem. With a small knife score each half 5mm (¼") from the edge, remove the flesh and roughly chop. Brush the insides of the aubergine halves with 1–2 tbsp of the olive oil, place on a metal tray and bake in the pre-heated oven for 25 minutes.

To prepare the risotto, measure a further 4 tbsp of oil in a large, heavy saucepan, add the onions and soften without colouring. Stir in the remainder from the aubergines, the garlic, ginger and rice until evenly coated with the cooking juices. Add the vegetable stock, bring to a simmer and cook uncovered for 15 minutes. Stir in the vinegar, cover and leave to stand for 5 minutes.

To make the spicy tomato sauce, heat the tomato pulp in a small saucepan, then stir in the coriander, cumin, thyme and cayenne pepper. Pre-heat a moderate grill. Spoon the risotto into the aubergine halves, scatter with pine nuts, top with grated Parmesan cheese, and brown under the grill. Spoon the tomato sauce on to four large plates, position two halves of aubergine on to the sauce, decorate with sprigs of fresh basil and serve.

Spinach And Macaroni Pie

Serves 4
Per serving:
Kcals   245
Fat   9.7g
Fibre   6.8g
300g (11oz) dried wholewheat macaroni
450g (1lb) fresh spinach or 225g (8oz) block of frozen spinach, thawed
50ml (2fl oz) skimmed milk
1 medium onion, chopped
3 cloves garlic, crushed
small piece root ginger, grated
100g (4oz) wholewheat breadcrumbs
50g (2oz) Parmesan cheese, grated
25g (1oz) sesame seeds

Pre-heat the oven to 190°C/375°F/gas mark 5 .

Cook the macaroni according to the instructions on the packet. Rinse in cold water to stop the cooking process and drain. If using fresh spinach, wash it and chop it into small pieces. Cook the fresh or frozen spinach in boiling water for 2–3 minutes. Place the spinach in a large mixing bowl. Add the milk, onion, garlic and grated ginger root to season. Stir in the cooked macaroni and transfer to a baking dish. Mix together the breadcrumbs, Parmesan cheese and sesame seeds. Sprinkle liberally over the macaroni mixture. Bake in the oven for 20–25 minutes or until the breadcrumbed topping is crisp and golden.

Stuffed Mushrooms with Hummous and Fresh Herbs

Serves 4
Per serving:
Kcals   529
Fat   9.0g
Fibre   5.2g

The upside-down caps of large button mushrooms provide the ideal resting place for hummous. Serve these mushrooms as an informal starter or lunchtime meal with a salad.

8 medium to large button mushrooms
1 tbsp olive oil
1 tbsp lemon juice
580g (1¼lb) low-fat hummous (see recipe page 83)
Salad:
1 curly green lettuce

100g (4oz) sugar snap peas, topped and tailed
100g (4oz) baby sweetcorn
1 small bunch fresh parsley, chopped
Dressing:
4 tbsp olive oil
2 tsp lemon juice
salt

Pre-heat a moderate grill. Snap off the mushroom stems from their bases (save for another recipe or salad) then arrange on a foil-lined tray. Combine 1 tbsp of the olive oil with the lemon juice, brush over the mushroom bases and grill for 6–8 minutes. Allow to cool. Spoon the hummous into the mushroom bases, then spread into tall cone shapes with a table knife. Mask one side of the hummous with freshly chopped parsley, spoon the paprika into a small sieve and dust the other side of the hummous. Top each mushroom with an olive and serve with the salad of curly lettuce, baby sweetcorn and parsley dressed with olive oil, lemon juice and a touch of salt.

Vegetable Stir-fry with Cashew Nuts and Rice Noodles FC (C)

Serves 4
Per serving:

Kcals	253
Fat	13.5g
Fibre	3.4g

200g (7oz) baby sweetcorn
200g (7oz) mange-tout
1 red or yellow pepper
2 courgettes
1 tbsp sesame oil
50g (2oz) cashew nuts
1 tbsp sesame seeds
200g (7oz) rice noodles
1–2 tbsp soy sauce

Prepare and chop or slice the vegetables and stir-fry in the sesame oil. Add the broken cashew nuts and sesame seeds. Cook the rice noodles, drain and add to the stir-fry together with the soy sauce, according to taste. Serve immediately.

Wild Mushroom Risotto FC (C)

Serves 4
Per serving:

Kcals	164
Fat	7.2g
Fibre	4.1g

1 onion, chopped

1–2 cloves garlic, crushed
1 tbsp olive oil
450g (1lb) mixed mushrooms, shiitake, chestnut, brown, cep, etc.
225g (8oz) wholegrain easy-cook rice or arborio risotto rice
750ml (1¼ pts) fresh vegetable stock, or additive-free stock cube such as Kallo
2 tbsp parsley, freshly grated
25g (1oz) Parmesan cheese **(P)**

In a medium-sized saucepan, sauté the onion and garlic in the oil until softened but not browned. Add the sliced mushrooms and cook for another 2 minutes. Stir in the rice and continue cooking for a further 2 minutes.

Add approximately 150ml (¼pt) of the stock and cook, stirring often over a low/medium heat. Continue until the rice has absorbed all the stock and is creamy and just tender. Stir in the parsley and serve sprinkled with grated or slivered Parmesan cheese, unless you are food combining.

MEAT

Beef Satay with a Hot Peanut Dip

Serves 4
Per serving:

Kcals	421g
Fat	15.6g
Fibre	2.9g

I've adapted this delicious dish to be lower in calories than usual. Peanuts combine well with warm spicy flavours to make these delicious skewers of lean beef. Beef satay are tastiest when cooked on a summer barbecue, although they are also good when grillled. This recipe can be adapted to use the same quantity of chicken breast, lean pork or Quorn for vegetarians.

300g (12oz) sirloin, trimmed of any fat
Marinade and dip:
50g (2oz) smooth peanut butter
1 clove garlic, crushed
150ml (5fl oz) low-fat yoghurt
juice of ½ lemon
2 tsp anchovy sauce
½ tsp chilli sauce
2 tsp caster sugar
400g (14oz) long-grain rice
Green salad:
3 little gem lettuces
1 curly head lettuce
¼ cucumber, sliced
1 bunch spring onions, chopped

1 small green pepper, de-seeded and sliced
Dressing:
2 tsp olive oil
2 tsp lemon juice or balsamic vinegar
pinch of salt

Slice the steak into 1cm (0.5") ribbons. Thread the steak zig-zag fashion on to eight 15cm (6") bamboo skewers and lay on a plate or tray. To make the marinade, combine all of the ingredients in a food processor or beat together until smooth. Spoon a third of the marinade over the beef and leave for at least half an hour, longer if you have time. Place the remainder of the sauce in a bowl to dip in to. Cook the rice according to packet instrucions, then wash and prepare the salad. Pre-heat a moderate grill or light a barbecue and let the coals settle to a steady glow. Grill or barbecue the beef skewers for 6–8 minutes turning once. Arrange two skewers per person on a portion of rice, dress the salad with olive oil, lemon juice and a sprinkling of salt. Serve with a bowl of dipping sauce.

Chicken and Pasta Shell Salad

Serves 4
Per serving:

Kcals	244
Fat	8.0g
Fibre	3.5g

This sumptuous salad is great way of using up leftover chicken and pasta and can be thrown together in seconds.

350g (12oz) wholemeal pasta shells
1 tbsp olive oil
225g (8oz) cold cooked chicken
2 small red and yellow peppers
25 g (1oz) pitted green or black olives
2 tbsp low-calorie mayonnaise
1 tsp Worcestershire sauce
1 tbsp balsamic or white wine vinegar
salt and freshly ground pepper
basil leaves to garnish

If you don't have any leftover pasta, cook and drain some wholemeal pasta shells and put into a large bowl. Add a few drops of olive oil, toss and allow to cool. Meanwhile, cut the chicken into bite-size pieces and mix together with all the other ingredients, except the pasta, in a salad bowl. When the pasta is cooked, add it to the salad bowl, season to taste and garnish with basil leaves.

Chicken with Peppers FC (P)

Serves 8
Per serving:
Kcals   417
Fat   17.8g
Fibre   2.0g
1.5kg (3lb) chicken, cut into serving pieces
3 large peppers, red, yellow or green, chopped and sliced
175g (6oz) shallots, finely sliced
1 tbsp dried chilli (optional)
100ml (4fl oz) white wine or chicken stock
salt and freshly ground black pepper
2 tbsp fresh parsley

Remove all the skin from the chicken and cut off any fat. Heat half the oil in a saucepan, add the chicken and brown on both sides. Then add the shallots, peppers, chilli and garlic to the pan with the remainder of the oil and cook until the peppers are soft. Add the wine or chicken stock and simmer until the liquid has reduced by half. Season to taste, cover the pan and simmer for about 25–30 minutes, stirring occasionally, until the chicken is cooked. Add the parsley and serve with rice or new potatoes, or neutral vegetables or salad if you are food combining.

Grilled Chicken Salad Louisiana

Serves 4
Per serving:
Kcals   311
Fat   14.9g
Fibre   7.7g
4 sweetcorn cobs
2 free-range boneless chicken breasts
4 rashers unsmoked back bacon (extra lean with all the fat cut off)
2 ripe bananas, peeled and halved
1 curly head lettuce
3 little gem lettuces
1 bunch watercress
12 cherry tomatoes
salt and freshly ground black pepper
Dressing:
2 tbsp groundnut (peanut) or vegetable oil
1 tbsp white wine vinegar
1 tsp maple syrup
2 tsp mustard

Pre-heat a moderate grill or light a barbecue and let the coals settle to a steady glow. Bring a large saucepan of salted water to the boil, shuck – remove the husks – and trim the corn cobs, then cook for 20 minutes. Slash the chicken breasts through 3 or 4 times with a sharp knife, season well and brush with oil. Grill or barbecue the chicken for 15 minutes, turning once, then grill the bacon for 8–10 minutes. Brush the bananas with oil and grill these for around 5 minutes, turning once. To make the dressing, combine all the ingredients in a screw-top jar, add 1 tbsp of water and shake well. Wash and dry the lettuce leaves, toss with the dressing and distribute between four large plates. Slice the chicken and arrange over the salad with the bacon, banana and the cherry tomatoes. Serve with the corn cobs.

Lamb and Bean Ragout FC (P)

Serves 6

Per serving:

Kcals	237
Fat	14g
Fibre	4.0g

The aromatic juniper berries in this delicious dish add a distinctive flavour that works well with the lamb and leeks.

100g (4oz) dried kidney beans, soaked overnight
1 tsp vegetable oil
1 large breast of lamb, trimmed and cut into chunks
450g (1lb) leeks, washed, trimmed and sliced
1 bay leaf
450ml (15fl oz) lamb stock
2 cloves of garlic, crushed
12 juniper berries
salt and pepper to season

Cook the kidney beans for ten minutes in boiling water, simmer for a further 30 minutes and drain. Meanwhile heat the oil in a large frying-pan or casserole dish and fry the lamb until browned. Add the leeks, beans, bay leaf, stock, garlic, juniper berries and seasoning. Bring to the boil, cover and simmer slowly for between 1 and 1 1/4 hours. Season to taste and serve with rice or new potatoes, or neutral vegetables or salad if you are food combining.

Lamb Paprika FC (P)

Serves 6

Per serving:

Kcals	256
Fat	13g
Fibre	3.0g

Delicious and simple.

1 tbsp olive oil
8 best-end neck chops, fat trimmed

2 medium onions, skinned and chopped
450g (1lb) tomatoes, skinned, quartered and seeded
225g (8oz) carrots, chopped
1 tbsp chopped parsley
1 heaped tsp paprika
salt and pepper to season
150ml (5fl oz) natural low-fat yoghurt

Heat the oil in a large frying-pan and brown the chops on both sides. Add the onions and carrots and fry until softened. Then add the tomatoes, parsley, paprika and seasoning. Bring to the boil, cover and simmer until tender for about half an hour. Then slowly stir in the yoghurt, stirring continuously, season to taste and serve with rice or new potatoes, or neutral vegetables or salad if you are food combining.

Lemon Chicken FC (P)

Serves 4
Per serving:
Kcals   300
Fat   22.9g
Fibre   0.1g
peel and juice of 1 lemon
1 onion
1 tbsp (15ml) olive oil
1 sprig of tarragon
25g (1oz) butter
freshly ground black pepper and sea salt
1 small free-range chicken

Pre-heat oven to 220°C/425°F/gas mark 7.

Make the stuffing with the lemon peel, the onion, the sprig of tarragon, butter, some freshly ground black pepper and a little salt. Stuff the chicken. Squeeze the juice from the lemon and use it to coat the outside of the chicken and add some salt and pepper.

Place the chicken on parchment baking paper with a thin covering of olive oil. Bring up the sides of the baking paper to form a loose parcel and wrap this in an outer sheet of foil.

Place in the oven for 20 minutes per lb plus 10–20 minutes extra. Halfway through cooking, remove the chicken from the oven and baste thoroughly. Open the top of the parcel for the last ten minutes of cooking to allow the chicken to brown. Serve with steamed vegetables or salad.

Light Frankfurter Salad with a Mustard and Caraway Dressing

Serves 4
Per serving:
Kcals   395
Fat   20.5g
Fibre   4.5g

700g (1¹/₂lb) new potatoes, scrubbed
3 free-range eggs
350g (12oz) light low-fat frankfurters
1 butterhead, batavian or endive lettuce
225g (8oz) young spinach leaves
salt and freshly ground black pepper

Dressing:
2 tbsp safflower or groundnut (peanut) oil
1 tbsp olive oil
1 tbsp white wine vinegar
2 tbsp mustard
1 tsp caraway seeds

Cover the potatoes with cold water, bring to the boil with a pinch of salt and cook for 20 minutes. Drain, cover and keep warm. Hard-boil the eggs for 12 minutes. Place in cold water, shell and cut into quarters. Place the low-fat frankfurters in a saucepan, cover with boiling water and heat them through. Combine the dressing ingredients in a screw-top jar and shake well. Wash and dry the salad leaves, moisten with half the dressing and distribute between four large plates. Drain the potatoes, cut them in half and place them with the drained frankfurters in a bowl. Cover the potatoes and frankfurters with the remainder of the dressing, then arrange over the salad leaves. Finish with sections of hard-boiled egg, season with salt and pepper and serve.

Mild Lamb Korma

Serves 8
Per serving:
Kcals   241
Fat   13.6g
Fibre   1.0g

Eastern cuisine has so much to offer our taste-buds, but the dishes available in Indian restaurants tend to be very high in fat and calories. I have adapted this authentic Indian recipe for lamb korma so that it has all of the taste, but only half the fat.

25g (1oz) butter
1 large onion, skinned and thinly sliced
2 cloves garlic, crushed
2.5cm (1") piece fresh root ginger, peeled, finely chopped

1 tbsp coriander seeds
6 green cardamoms (optional)
900g (2lb) boneless lamb fillet, trimmed and cut into cubes
2 tsp ground turmeric
finely grated rind and juice of one lemon
50g (2oz) ground almonds
salt and pepper to season
200ml (7fl oz) low-fat yoghurt
grated lemon and flaked almonds to garnish

Heat the butter in a saucepan or large frying-pan, add the onion, garlic and ginger and fry gently for about ten minutes, stirring often.

Meanwhile, grind the coriander seeds and cardamoms in a small electric mill or by hand with a pestle and mortar. Once ground, add to the pan and mix well. Fry for 2 minutes while stirring constantly. Then add the lamb to the pan a few pieces at a time and mix in the turmeric and lemon juice. Season to taste, cover and simmer gently for about 50 minutes, until the lamb is tender, turning the meat frequently.

Finally, slowly add the yoghurt to the pan, stirring continuously and heat it through. Add more salt and pepper if required and sprinkle with flaked almonds and grated lemon peel.

Pork and Pasta Stir-fry

Serves 6
Per serving:

Kcals	246
Fat	10 g
Fibre	2.5 g

The apple and cider bring out the sweet taste of the pork in this delicious, low-calorie stir-fry.

450g (1lb) pork tenderloin
75g (3oz) fat-trimmed bacon, rinded and chopped
225g (8oz) onions, skinned and finely sliced
1 small apple, diced
1 level tbsp wholegrain mustard
100ml (4fl oz) dry cider
1 garlic clove, skinned and crushed
1 tbsp olive or sunflower oil
salt and pepper
175g (6oz) green beans, topped, tailed and halved
1 red pepper, seeded and cut into strips
75g (3oz) wholemeal pasta shells
4 tbsp stock
1 tbsp soy sauce

Cut the pork into long, thin strips, discarding any skin and excess fat and put in a bowl with the bacon, onions, apple, mustard, cider, garlic, oil and seasoning. Mix all the ingredients together thoroughly, cover and leave to marinate in the fridge for an hour or so. Meanwhile, boil the green beans and pepper together for 2 minutes in boiling water and cook the pasta until *al dente* for about 8 minutes. Drain and toss with a few drops of olive oil to prevent it sticking together. Drain the marinade juices from the meat, onions and apples and put to one side. Heat 2 tablespoons of oil in a frying-pan, add meat, onions and apple and stir-fry for about 4 minutes on a high heat. Meanwhile put the beans, pepper and pasta into a saucepan with the stock, seasoning, soy sauce and marinade. Bring to the boil, stir and then simmer for about 5 minutes until hot and serve with the piping hot stir-fry.

Sopa de Picadillo

Serves 4
Per serving:

Kcals	306
Fat	16.2g
Fibre	1.4g

At the end of a long hot day, I sometimes turn to this thick main course broth made with potato, carrot and strips of gammon. What appeals most is that this Spanish meal is as easy to make as it is to eat. The dish is ideally made with short-grain risotto rice, but you can also use ordinary long-grain.

> *3 tbsp olive oil*
> *1 medium onion, chopped*
> *1 medium carrot, peeled and diced*
> *1 medium potato, peeled and diced*
> *1 gammon steak, unsmoked*
> *150g (5oz) risotto or long-grain rice*
> *900ml (1¹/2pts) chicken stock* ✱
> *2 tbsp lemon juice*
> *salt and pepper*
> *2 tbsp freshly chopped mint*
> ✱ I use additive free stock cubes because they contain no artificial flavouring or preservative. Look out for the Kallo brand in leading supermarkets.

Place the oil, onion, carrot and potato in a large saucepan and soften for about 6–8 minutes without colouring. Cut the gammon into short strips, stir into the vegetables and cook briefly. Stir in the rice so that the grains are coated evenly with the cooking juices. Pour in the chicken stock and simmer uncovered for about 20 minutes. Sharpen the broth with lemon juice, season to taste, ladle into shallow soup plates and serve scattered with freshly chopped mint.

Spicy Lamb-stuffed Courgettes

Serves 4
Per serving:
Kcals   170
Fat   9.0g
Fibre   1.3g
2 large courgettes
1 onion, chopped
1 tbsp olive oil
225g (8oz) minced lamb
1 tbsp tomato purée
1 tsp cumin
1 tsp currrants
50g (2oz) cooked rice

Halve the courgettes, brush the cut edge with a little oil and place on a baking-tray in a medium hot oven for 10–15 minutes until softened. Scoop out the middle flesh, leaving a good bit on the skins to form the 'shells'. Sauté the onion and clove of garlic in the oil, add the lamb and brown. Add the tomato purée, cumin, currants, rice, and the cooked courgette flesh. Moisten with a little water and pack into the courgette halves. Cover with foil and bake in a medium-hot oven for 15–20 minutes.

Spicy Rubbed Chicken FC (P)

Serves 4
Per serving:
Kcals   126
Fat   5 g
Fibre   0.1 g

This delicious recipe is very quick and easy to put together and is a perfect dish for effortless entertaining.

1 chicken, cut into large pieces
1 tbsp lemon juice
1 tbsp extra virgin olive oil
1 cup (8fl oz) oregano leaves, finely chopped
1 cup (8fl oz) rosemary leaves, finely chopped
1 cup (8fl oz) thyme leaves, finely chopped
salt and pepper to season

Wash the chicken pieces and pat dry. Whisk the lemon juice and olive oil in a large bowl, add the chicken and marinate in the fridge for an hour. Mix together the oregano, rosemary, thyme and salt and pepper in a bowl and drench each piece of chicken so that it is evenly coated with the marinade. Then simply grill the chicken for 20–25 minutes until cooked through. To test the chicken, pierce it with a knife and if the juice runs clear it is fully cooked. Serve with rice or new potatoes, or neutral vegetables or salad if you are food combining.

Steak Salad

Serves 4

Per serving:

Kcals	420
Fat	17.2g
Fibre	7.9g

The flavours that make up this nourishing salad have been borrowed from a New York sandwich called 'Po' Boy'. For this salad version, fresh ingredients are laid out on a plate and enjoyed with a basket of crispy French bread.

4 x100g (4oz) sirloin steaks, trimmed of all fat
1 lettuce
1 bunch watercress
3 large spring onions
4 canned baby artichoke hearts, halved
100g (4oz) button mushrooms, sliced
4 tomatoes, quartered
12 large green olives
4 large dill pickles, sliced
salt and freshly ground black pepper
1 French baguette stick

Dressing:

4 tbsp olive oil, plus a little extra for cooking the meat
1 tbsp white wine vinegar
1 tsp mustard
2 tsp horseradish sauce

Pre-heat a moderate grill, or light a barbecue and let the coals settle to a steady glow. Season the steaks with pepper, moisten with olive oil and cook for 6–8 minutes, turning once until cooked as you like them. Cover and leave the meat to rest in a warm place.

To make the dressing, measure ingredients into a screw-top jar and shake. Wash the salad leaves and dry. Place salad in a large bowl, slice the spring onions lengthways and add with the artichoke hearts and mushrooms. Add the dressing and toss well. Distribute the tossed salad between four large plates, slice the warm steak diagonally and position over the salad. Scatter the tomatoes, olives and pickles over the salad, season with salt and serve with a basket of crispy French bread.

Summer Chicken Stir-fry FC (P)

Serves 4

Per serving:

Kcals	288
Fat	9.0g
Fibre	7.0g

This tasty stir-fry is full of delicious vegetables and is extremely quick and easy to make. The vegetables should only be lightly cooked so that they stay crunchy and maintain most of their vitamins.

2 chicken breasts, cubed
1 large onion, sliced
3 carrots, peeled and sliced
50g (2oz) tinned beansprouts
1 tbsp olive oil
1 red and yellow pepper, sliced
50g (2oz) mushrooms, peeled and sliced
50g (2oz) baby sweetcorn
50g (2oz) tinned bamboo shoots
50g (2oz) mange-touts
salt, pepper and soy sauce to season

Heat the oil in a wok or large frying-pan and cook the chicken and onion for about five minutes until the chicken is cooked through. Then add the carrots and cook for a minute before adding the other ingredients. The mange-touts should be added last of all so that they stay nice and crunchy. Finally season to taste with salt, pepper and soy sauce and serve with rice noodles, unless you are food combining.

Summer Lamb Hotpot

Serves 6
Per serving:

Kcals	460
Fat	20g
Fibre	5.0g

This hearty hotpot is great for Sunday lunches or those cooler summer evenings and is full of flavour.

225g (8 oz) haricot beans
25ml (1fl oz) olive oil
225g (8oz) pieces of lean bacon, cut into 1cm (1/2")pieces trimmed of fat
2 cloves garlic, crushed
275g (10oz) sliced onions
225g (8oz) carrots, diced
100g (4oz) celery, diced
100g (4oz) fennel, diced
900g (2lb) lamb (leg or shoulder), trimmed of fat
1 x 400g (14oz) tin of tomatoes
bouquet garni – made up of thyme, parsley, rosemary
salt and freshly ground pepper
parsley to garnish

Soak the beans in water overnight. Heat the olive oil in a casserole dish and fry the bacon until crisp, before adding the garlic and onions. When the onion and garlic has softened, add the diced carrots, celery and fennel, cover, lower the heat and steam for a few minutes.

Meanwhile cut the lamb into bite-sized chunks and brown in a little olive oil in a separate pan. Then add the lamb, chopped tomatoes and drained beans to the vegetables and season with salt and pepper. Finally, add the bouquet garni, bring to the boil, cover and simmer for 1 to 1¹/₂ hours. Garnish with chopped parsley and serve with a portion of rice.

Thai Chicken with Prawn Soup FC (P)

Serves 4
Per serving:

Kcals	259
Fat	15g
Fibre	0.4g

This soup has a spicy and unusually pungent flavour.

2 boned and skinned chicken breasts
2cm (1") fresh ginger, peeled and chopped
1 stem lemon grass, shredded
1 clove garlic, halved
2 lime leaves, optional ✳
¹/₂ chicken stock cube
100g (4oz) coconut milk ♠
3 tbsp fish sauce (see page 120) or water
225g (8oz) tiger prawn tails, raw or cooked, peeled
¹/₂ tsp chilli sauce
2 tsp sugar
3 tbsp lime juice
2 spring onions, green part only, sliced to garnish
1 small bunch fresh coriander

✳ Fresh lime leaves have a rich pungent flavour and are often sold in packs of Thai herbs and spices in leading supermarkets.

♠ Coconut milk is packed with fat, but the small amount used here is essential for the flavour of the dish. You can find it in larger supermarkets and delicatessens. You can also use coconut water, which is much lower in fat.

Place the chicken breasts, ginger, lemon grass, garlic, lime leaves and stock cube in a saucepan, add 600ml (1 pint) of water, bring to the boil and simmer for 10 minutes. Remove any scum that rises to the surface, then strain the liquid into a clean saucepan. Slice the chicken and discard the spices. Add the coconut milk and fish sauce to the strained liquid and bring to a simmer. Return the chicken to the liquid, add the prawns, chilli sauce and lime juice, and simmer for 2–3 minutes. Ladle the soup into four bowls and scatter with spring onion and coriander.

Thai Marinaded Chicken and Vegetable Kebabs FC (P)

Serves 4
Per serving:
Kcals   247
Fat   9.0g
Fibre   2.8g

This is another excellent idea for the barbecue and can also be made with tofu
or Quorn for vegetarians.

450g (1lb) chicken or turkey breast fillet, cut into cubes
*750g (1¹/₂lb) vegetables (courgette, mange-tout, yellow or red pepper, baby
    sweetcorn, etc.)*

Marinade:
1 tbsp olive oil
1 tbsp clear honey
2 limes, juice and grated rind
2 cloves garlic, crushed
2cm (1") fresh ginger, grated or chopped
1 stalk lemon grass, chopped
1 red chilli
2 tbsp fresh coriander, chopped

Mix all the marinade ingredients together and pour over the chicken, cover and
leave to marinate in the fridge for at least 2 hours. Prepare the vegetables, cut into
small chunks and add to the chicken. Mix and coat evenly with the marinade.
Thread on to skewers and cook them on the barbecue or under a medium-hot grill.

Turkey Breasts with Ratatouille FC (P)

Serves 4
Per serving:
Kcals   202
Fat   5.9g
Fibre   4.2g

1 onion, chopped
1 clove garlic, crushed
2 large courgettes, sliced
1 tsp mixed herbs
1 tbsp olive oil
1 aubergine, sliced
2 peppers (red, green or yellow), chopped
450g (1lb) chopped tomatoes
4 turkey breasts

A quicker method for this recipe is to open a can of ratatouille!

Otherwise sauté the chopped onion and crushed garlic in half the olive oil,
add the aubergine, courgettes and peppers and cook for a few minutes before

adding the tomatoes and the mixed herbs. Cook until soft. Meanwhile, grill the turkey breasts, brushed with the remaining oil and serve with the ratatouille.

FISH

Cod Kebabs with Basil Sauce FC (P)

Serves 4
Per serving:

Kcals   333
Fat   10.7g
Fibre   1.1g

1kg (2lb) chunky cod steaks, skinned and boned
1 red and 1 yellow pepper
juice and grated zest of 1 lemon
2 tbsp sunflower oil
salt and pepper to season
Sauce:
1 clove garlic, crushed
2–3 tbsp freshly chopped basil leaves
3 tbsp low-fat fromage frais
salt and pepper

Wash the fish and cut into cubes. Scorch the peppers over a gas flame or under a hot grill until the skins are black, then peel and slice the peppers, removing all the seeds. Mix together the lemon juice, oil and seasoning in a basin, add the fish and pepper pieces and marinate for 20 minutes.

Meanwhile, you can make the sauce. Mix the crushed garlic, chopped basil and fromage frais together in a saucepan, season and heat very gently, stirring all the time. When the sauce thickens to a creamy consistency, remove from the heat and keep warm. Do not let it boil. To cook the fish, heat the grill until very hot and oil the grill rack. Lightly oil the kebab skewers. Thread the cubes of fish and pieces of pepper alternately on the skewers and cook under the grill for about 4 minutes, turning occasionally and basting with the marinade mixture. Serve immediately on a bed of rice (unless food combining) and pour the basil sauce over each kebab.

Fast Fish Risotto

Serves 2
Per serving:

Kcals   290
Fat   14g
Fibre   3.5g

This is a good way of using up leftover bits of fish and/or rice. Whole Earth make tinned brown rice which I use a lot as it tastes good and is a great time-saver.

100g (4oz) fresh oily fish (e.g. mackerel or herring)
1 onion, peeled and finely chopped
1 tbsp olive oil
6 heaped tbsps cooked brown rice
150g (5oz) frozen peas
1 tbsp freshly chopped basil and parsley

If using fresh fish, cook under a hot grill for about 5 minutes, turning once. Allow to cool slightly, then flake the fish flesh into large pieces. Alternatively, open a can of tuna. Heat the oil in a large frying-pan and lightly fry the onion. Add the fish, rice and peas. Stir continuously to prevent the mixture sticking to the sides of the frying-pan while heating through for about 3 minutes to cook the peas. Garnish with the chopped basil or parsley before serving.

Fish and Fennel Risotto

Serves 4
Per serving:

Kcals	251
Fat	3.7g
Fibre	4.0g

This is a favourite of mine as it has a delicate flavour, yet is really filling.

1 tsp sunflower oil
1 onion, finely chopped
2 large fennel bulbs
grated rind and juice of one lemon
225g (8oz) long-grain brown rice
600ml (20fl oz) boiling water
450g (1lb) fillets cod or coley
100g (4oz) spinach or watercress, chopped
225g (8oz) fresh tomatoes, chopped
50g (2oz) freshly grated Parmesan cheese
pinch of salt

Gently soften the onion in the oil in a large pan until it is translucent, but not browned.

Meanwhile, remove the tough outer skin of the fennel, trim the bases and stalks, and slice the bulbs into chunky strips. Keep the delicate leafy fronds to use as a garnish. Add the fennel and grated lemon rind to the onion and cook for a further 2 minutes. Add the rice, mix in well, then pour in the boiling water. Return to the boil, cover and cook on the lowest possible heat for 30 minutes until nearly all the water is absorbed.

While the rice is cooking, cut the fish fillets into small pieces and add to the rice, stirring carefully so as not to break it up. Continue to cook for a further 5 minutes before adding the other ingredients to the risotto. Stir carefully and cook for 2 more minutes. Season to taste with a pinch of salt and the lemon juice. Serve immediately and garnish with the fennel fronds.

Fillets of Sole with Pink Grapefruit and Lime

Serves 4
Per serving:

Kcals	358
Fat	6.1g
Fibre	5.2g

Pink grapefruits have a gentle sweetness that complements the richness of the sole prepared here in a not-too-creamy sauce. Fillets of plaice can be used instead of sole.

450g (1lb) fillets of lemon sole, skin removed
salt and cayenne pepper to season
400g (14oz) long-grain rice
1 pink grapefruit
350g (12oz) new carrots, scraped
350g (12oz) broccoli, cut into florets
15g (¹/₂oz) butter
juice of ¹/₂ lemon
45ml (3fl oz) dry vermouth or white wine
2 tsp cornflour
2 tbsp low-fat crème fraîche
4 slices lime to garnish

To season the fish, combine a pinch of cayenne pepper with 3–4 pinches of fine salt. Sprinkle over the fish then fold the fillets in half so that the whitest side is uppermost and set aside. Put the rice on to cook according to instructions. To segment the grapefruit, remove the top and bottom with a sharp knife, stand on one end, then pare away the skin and pith by cutting down the curved side of the fruit. Remove segments from the grapefruit by working the knife in between the sections. Set aside.

Bring a kettle of water to the boil and put the carrots and broccoli in two separate saucepans, each with a pinch of salt, cover with water and cook both for 6 minutes. Put the butter and lime juice in a large shallow pan. Lay the folded fillets over the top, then pour in the vermouth and 75 ml (3fl oz) water. Bring to a gentle simmer, cover and cook for not more than one minute. Lift the fillets out on to a warm plate. Mix the cornflour with 1 tbsp of cold water, add to the cooking juices, stir and simmer to thicken. Add the crème fraîche, grapefruit segments and season to taste with salt and cayenne pepper. Arrange the fillets on to 4 plates, spoon on the sauce and serve with carrots, broccoli and rice.

Fishy Jacket Potatoes

Serves 4
Per serving:
Kcals   279
Fat   6.0g
Fibre   3.0g

This is a baked potato with a difference! The combination of fish, herbs, garlic and cheese is very tasty, low in fat and amazingly filling.

350g (12oz) cooked fish
4 large baked potatoes
175g (6oz) cheddar cheese, grated
2 cloves of garlic, crushed
2 tbsp parsley or coriander, finely chopped
1–2 tbsp skimmed milk
salt and ground pepper to season

Remove all skin and bones from fish and flake it gently with a fork. Cut the potatoes in half lengthways and scoop out the flesh. Mash it finely forking in 100g (4oz) of grated cheese, the garlic, chopped parsley or coriander and the milk, until the mixture is smooth. Now carefully fork in the flaked fish and season to taste with pepper. Pile the mixture back into the potato shells, scatter with the remaining 50g (2oz) cheese and bake in the oven for 20 minutes at 400°F/200°C/gas mark 6.

To Microwave: Prick the potatoes all over with a fork, cook on high for 15 minutes and turn halfway through cooking. Stuff the potatoes as above, then cook on high for 2–3 minutes. Deliciously simple.

Grilled Salmon Steaks with Fennel FC (P)

Serves 4
Per serving:
Kcals   315
Fat   23.8g
Fibre   0.3g

Salmon always makes a delicious summer meal and is surprisingly filling. The aniseed taste of the fennel seeds works perfectly with the delicate taste of the fish.

juice of 1 lemon
3 tbsp (45g) chopped fresh fennel
1 tsp fennel or dill seeds
2 tbsp olive or sunflower oil
4 salmon steaks of the same thickness (about 500g/1.5lb total)
salt and freshly ground pepper to season
lemon wedges and fresh dill to garnish

Mix together the lemon juice, chopped fennel and fennel seeds with the olive oil in a bowl. Add the salmon steaks and thoroughly coat with the marinade. Sprinkle with salt and pepper, cover with clingfilm and place in the fridge for a couple of hours. Then re-heat the grill, arrange the fish in one layer on a shallow baking tray or ovenproof dish with half the marinade. Grill about 10cm (4") from the heat source for 6–8 minutes, turning halfway through, until both sides are browned. Serve hot and garnish with the lemon wedges.

Halibut with Watercress Sauce FC (P)

Serves 4
Per serving:

Kcals	434
Fat	17.9g
Fibre	1.0g

Halibut is ideal for baking because it can be cut like a steak, has a firm texture and doesn't fall apart as you transfer it to a plate. Alternatively use hoki, an inexpensive alternative from New Zealand.

1 small onion, finely chopped
150ml (¼ pint) dry white wine
1kg (approx. 2lb) halibut steaks
2 tbsp olive oil
100g (4oz) watercress, chopped
1 tsp smooth mustard
salt and pepper

Pre-heat the oven to 230°C/450°F/gas mark 8.

Place the onions and white wine in a casserole dish or stainless steel baking pan (with a lid). Lay the halibut steaks on top and drizzle with olive oil. Cover and bake in the pre-heated oven for about 15–20 minutes until almost cooked through. Move the fish to a hot serving dish and cover with a lid or a piece of foil to keep warm. Transfer the cooking juices to a small saucepan, add the chopped watercress and boil on a high heat for about a minute. Use a hand-held blender (or transfer to a food processor) to purée the sauce until smooth. Add the mustard, salt and pepper to taste and pour over the fish just before serving.

Jamaica Spiced Cod with a Tomato and Coriander Salsa

Serves 4
Per serving:

Kcals	412
Fat	9.6g
Fibre	3.7g

One of the most appealing qualities of fresh cod is that it can be put with hot fruity spices without masking its underlying flavour. You can also use hoki, a cheaper alternative.

4 x 175g (6oz) cod or hoki steaks
½ orange
2 tbsp black peppercorns

> 1 tbsp allspice berries
> 1/2 tsp salt
> 2 tbsp olive oil

Salsa:

> 4 ripe tomatoes
> 1 small onion, finely chopped
> 1 small bunch coriander, roughly chopped
> 750g (1½lb) new potatoes, scrubbed
> 350g (12oz) green beans, topped and tailed

Finely grate the orange zest into a small bowl. Add the peppercorns, allspice and salt, then crush coarsely with the back of a teaspoon. Alternatively grind the peppercorns and allspice coarsely in a peppermill and combine with the orange zest. Scatter the spice mixture over both sides of the fish, moisten with oil and set aside. Cover the potatoes with cold water, add a pinch of salt, bring to the boil and cook for 20 minutes.

To make the salsa, cut the tomatoes in half through the stem. Remove the stem from each half and chop roughly. Combine the onion and coriander, add a pinch of salt and set aside. Pre-heat a moderate grill and cook the fish for 12 minutes, turning once. Cover the beans with boiling water, add a pinch of salt and cook for 5 minutes. When the fish is cooked, serve with new potatoes, green beans and a spoonful of salsa on the side.

Nasi Goreng – Indonesian Pork and Prawn Rice

> Serves 4
> Per serving:

Kcals	521
Fat	21g
Fibre	6.9g

Nasi Goreng is the fast food of the Indonesian street market, made to order in a large wok. This recipe partners pork and prawns, and includes a lively mix of warm spices. Raw prawn tails offer an authentic flavour and can be found at the fish counters of larger supermarkets and high-quality fishmongers. Delicatessens and larger supermarkets also stock creamed coconut. It is very high in calories, so I've only used a tiny amount.

> 250g (9oz) long grain rice ✱ or 500g (18oz) cooked rice
> 3 free-range eggs
> 2 tbsp vegetable oil
> 2 cloves garlic, crushed
> 2cm (1") root ginger, peeled and chopped
> 1/2 tsp chilli paste
> 1/2 tsp turmeric
> 15g (1/2oz) creamed coconut
> 1 tsp sugar

2 tbsp lime juice
50ml (2fl oz) fish sauce ♠ or water
275g (10oz) lean pork or skinless chicken breasts, sliced
225g (8oz) raw or cooked prawn tails, peeled
175g (6oz) beansprouts
175g (6oz) Chinese leaves, shredded
175g (6oz) frozen peas
salt
1 small bunch coriander or basil, chopped to garnish

* Long grain rice is sold either part cooked, so-called easy cook or white grain, which has a natural stickiness. Ordinary white grain rice is best for flavour – better still look out for authentic Jasmin or Thai rices which have a gentle Basmati fragrance.

♠ Fish sauce is the South East Asian equivalent of soya sauce and is used to impart an addictive fish flavour to regional cooking. It is worth looking for, although you may have to go to a specialist food store to find it.

If starting with uncooked rice, put the measured amount in a saucepan, cover with 500ml (18fl oz) of boiling water and a pinch of salt. Stir once and simmer uncovered for 15 minutes, switch off the heat, cover and allow to stand for a further 5 minutes. If you happen to have the equivalent of 500g (18oz) of coooked rice, heat it through in a microwave (5 minutes at medium power) or position the rice in a wire sieve over a pan of simmering water, cover and heat through for 10–12 minutes.

To make the omelette garnish, beat the eggs in a bowl with a pinch of salt. Heat a non-stick frying-pan over a moderate heat, pour in the beaten egg and move it around with a spatula until it begins to set. When the eggs have set completely, turn the egg pancake on to a plate. Roll the pancake up tightly, cut into 1cm (0.5") ribbons, cover and set aside. Heat the oil, garlic, chilli and turmeric in a large wok and stir until the flavours combine (less than a minute), Add the creamed coconut, sugar, lime and the fish sauce or water. Stir in the pork and prawns and cook for 3–4 minutes. Toss in the beansprouts, Chinese leaves and peas with the spices, add the rice and stir-fry for 6–8 minutes, keeping it moving to prevent burning. Turn the Nasi Goreng out on to a large serving plate, lay the omelette strips over the top, scatter with coriander or basil and serve.

Prawn-filled Pitta Pockets

Serves 4
Per serving:

Kcals	203
Fat	2.0g
Fibre	3.0g

These fish pitta rolls are much lower in fat than ordinary pancakes and are really spicy. They look great and are perfect low-fat canapés for summer parties.

2 little gem lettuces, shredded
1 bunch spring onions, finely chopped
1/2 tbsp root ginger, very finely chopped
1 tbsp mint, finely chopped
1 tsp grated lemon zest
175g (6oz) peeled prawns
100g (4oz) low-fat fromage frais
salt and freshly ground pepper to season
4 wholemeal pitta breads

Mix together the shredded lettuce, spring onions, ginger, mint and lemon in a large bowl. Add the prawns and fromage frais and season with salt and freshly ground black pepper. Slice the pitta breads in half, spoon a generous amount of the salad mixture on a pitta bread half and roll it up (a bit like a stuffed pancake).

Prawn Kebabs with Herb Dressing FC (P)

Serves 2
Per serving:

Kcals	287
Fat	23.8g
Fibre	1.5g

You can also make these simple kebabs with chunks of chicken, Quorn or tofu.
Kebabs:

12 king-sized prawns
8 button mushrooms
1 medium courgette, sliced

Herb dressing:

3 tbsp olive oil or sunflower oil
1 clove garlic, crushed
juice of 1 lemon
1 sprig each of basil, parsley and tarragon, finely chopped

Thread the prawns, button mushrooms and sliced courgette on to wooden or metal skewers and place in a shallow dish. Mix the ingredients for the herb dressing together and pour over the threaded skewers. Cover and leave to marinade for 30 minutes, turning them occasionally.

Place under a medium-hot grill and cook for about 3 minutes, basting and turning them as they cook.

Salmon and Sweet Potato Pie with Wilted Greens

Serves 4
Per serving:

Kcals   306
Fat   18.5g
Fibre   4.1g

This dish is also a good way of using up leftover cold salmon or any other type of fish.

200g (8oz) fresh salmon steaks
1 tbsp fresh lemon juice
1 tbsp fresh dill, chopped
salt and black pepper
100g (4oz) wholewheat pasta shells, cooked and drained
1 tbsp olive oil
4fl oz skimmed milk
200g (8oz) cooked, mashed sweet potatoes
50g (2oz) toasted sunflower seeds
1 tsp olive oil for greasing baking dish
Greens:
350g (12oz) fresh spinach or spinach greens
1 tsp freshly grated ginger root
1 tsp soya or tamari sauce

Pre-heat the oven to 190°C/375°F/gas mark 5. Place the salmon in a baking dish, sprinkle with lemon juice, dill and salt and pepper to season. Cover and bake for 15 minutes, or until cooked. Flake the fish and set aside. Mix the skimmed milk and olive oil, stir in the sweet potatoes and mix well. Add the pre-cooked pasta, flaked salmon pieces and toasted sunflower seeds. Oil the baking dish to prevent the mixture from sticking. Pour the mixture into the dish, cover and bake in the oven for 20 minutes. Prepare the wilted greens by washing and trimming any tough stalks. Place in a steamer over a pan of boiling water, sprinkle with ginger root and lightly steam for 5–10 minutes. Alternatively, microwave until just softened. Remove from the pan, sprinkle with soya sauce and serve with the pie.

Salmon with Watercress Sauce

Serves 4
Per serving:

Kcals   243
Fat   17.6g
Fibre   1.0g

1 bunch watercress, chopped
1 bunch spring onions, chopped
1 tbsp olive oil

100ml vegetable stock
100g (4oz) low-fat soft cheese with garlic and herb seasoning
4 salmon fillets

Sauté the chopped onions and watercress in the oil, stirring frequently until softened, add the stock and simmer for 5 minutes. Liquidise the watercress mixture, add the soft cheese and whizz again if necessary. Meanwhile, heat the grill and cook the salmon skin side up for 2 minutes, turn over and continue to grill for 2–4 minutes depending on the thickness of the fish. Serve the salmon with the sauce.

Spiced Prawns FC (P)

Serves 6
Per serving:

Kcals	268
Fat	10.8g
Fibre	2.0g

3 tbsp olive oil
1 medium onion, finely chopped
1 stick celery, finely chopped
1 small red pepper, seeded and chopped
1 tbsp red wine vinegar or balsamic vinegar
1 x 400g (14oz) can plum tomatoes, chopped with their juice
salt and freshly ground pepper to season
1kg (2lb) fresh prawns
2–3 cloves garlic, finely chopped
3 tbsp chopped fresh parsley

Heat half the oil in a saucepan and cook the onion on a low heat until soft. Stir in the celery and chopped pepper, and cook for 5 minutes more. Raise the heat to medium high, and add the vinegar and tomatoes. Season with salt and pepper. Bring to the boil and cook for about 5 minutes. Then lower the heat, cover the pan and simmer for about 30 minutes until the vegetables are soft. Remove the sauce from the heat and purée it in a food processor or blender or alternatively, mash the sauce through a sieve.

Shell the prawns and de-vein them, by making a shallow incision with a small sharp knife down the centre of the back to disclose the long black vein. Remove the vein and discard.

Heat the remaining oil in a clean heavy saucepan and add the garlic and parsley. Cook over a moderate heat, stirring constantly, until the garlic is golden – but not brown. Then add the smooth tomato sauce and bring to the boil. Season to taste, stir in the prawns and bring to the boil again. Reduce the heat slightly and simmer until the prawns are pink, 6–8 minutes depending on their size. Remove from the heat and serve.

Sweet and Sour Sole

Serves 4
Per serving:

Kcals   234
Fat   2.0g
Fibre   2.0g

4 tbsp wholemeal flour
salt and freshly ground pepper to season
pinch of ground allspice
3–4 fillets of sole or any flat fish
6–8 tbsp olive oil
1 small onion, very finely sliced
4 tbsp dry white wine
4 tbsp white wine vinegar
1 small tin of pineapple chunks in water

Season the flour with the allspice, salt and pepper and use to coat the sole fillets. Then heat 3 tbsp of the oil in a heavy frying-pan. Cook the sole fillets a few at a time until golden, about 3 minutes on each side. Then using a slotted fish slice, transfer the fish fillets to a large shallow serving dish. Add the remaining oil to the saucepan then fry the onion over a low heat until golden. Mix in the wine, vinegar and pineapple chunks, bring to the boil and simmer for 4–5 minutes. Pour this sauce over the fish, cover with foil, and leave in a cool place for an hour or so (to allow the fish to absorb the sweet flavour of the sauce). Then simply reheat the dish and serve at room temperature.

Tuna and Sweetcorn Potato Cakes

Serves 4
Per serving:

Kcals   237
Fat   1.3g
Fibre   3.5g

750g (1¹/₂lb) potatoes
200g (7oz) can tuna (in brine)
200g (7oz) can sweetcorn
2 tbsp parsley
50g (2oz) flour or dried breadcrumbs
salt and pepper
1 lemon

This is a good way of using up leftover mashed potatoes. Otherwise cook and mash the potatoes, drain the tuna and sweetcorn and add to the potato, together with the chopped parsley and seasoning. Mix together and form into potato cakes, roll in a little flour or breadcrumbs and grill or ovenbake in a hot oven until golden brown and piping hot. Serve warm with lemon wedges.

Warm Cod Salad FC (P)

Serves 4
Per serving:

Kcals	164
Fat	5.0g
Fibre	4.0g

4 cod or coley steaks

Marinade:

1 tbsp sunflower or olive oil
300ml (10fl oz) dry white wine
300ml (10fl oz) white wine vinegar
2–4 fat cloves garlic, finely chopped and crushed
1 tsp soya sauce
grated rind and juice of 2 large oranges
grated rind and juice of 2 large lemons
1 tsp dried parsley, oregano and tarragon
freshly ground black pepper to season

Salad:

1 crisp lettuce or endive
1 radicchio lettuce
2 bunches watercress
6 spring onions, finely sliced
100g (4oz) button mushrooms, quartered
1 bunch radishes, sliced
1 tbsp fresh parsley or coriander, finely chopped, to garnish

Wash the cod steaks and pat dry with some kitchen towel. Heat a little oil in a frying-pan and lightly cook the steaks for two minutes on each side until cooked through. Carefully lift them out with a slotted spoon and put them in a heatproof glass dish suitable for marinating.

Add all the other marinade ingredients to the fishy juices in the pan and bring to simmering point. Continue to cook for five minutes. Then pour the hot marinade over the cod steaks and leave to cool. Cover the dish with cling-film and leave in a cool place to marinade for about four hours.

Then, when the four hours marinading time is nearly up, wash and shred the lettuce and radicchio, remove the stalks from the watercress and trim and slice the spring onions. Wash and thinly slice the courgettes, mushrooms and radishes and then mix all the vegetables together .

Remove the cod steaks from the marinade, and with a knife and fork ease the flakes off the bone. Pour the marinade juices into a saucepan, return to the heat and warm gently.

Separate the salad ingredients on to four plates and place a portion of flaked fish on top. Pour over a little of the warm juice from the marinade and garnish with the chopped parsley or coriander.

arm Seafood and Pasta Salad

Serves 4
Per serving:
Kcals   365
Fat   9.5g
Fibre   0.3g

2 cloves garlic, crushed
2cm (1") fresh ginger, grated
1 bunch spring onions, chopped
1 tbsp olive oil
3 tbsp white wine or stock
350g (12oz) mixed seafood, e.g. shrimps, clams, squid, etc.
2 tbsp chopped fresh herbs, e.g. dill, coriander, parsley, etc.
4 tbsp low-calorie dressing or mayonnaise
275g (10oz) fresh pasta, e.g linguine, tagliatelle
1 lemon or lime

Sauté the garlic, ginger and spring onions in the oil for 2–3 minutes until softened. Add the white wine or stock and allow to bubble for 2 minutes before adding the seafood. Cook for a further 2 minutes to heat through. Remove from the heat and stir in the herbs and low-calorie dressing. Meanwhile, cook the pasta and drain. Serve the pasta topped with the seafood and garnished with lemon or lime wedges.

ACCOMPANIMENTS

Tapenade FC (N)

Makes 175g (6oz)
Per 44g serving:
Kcals   130.4
Fat   14g
Fibre   0.9g

This rich olive paste from Provence can be used to coat fish fillets, chicken breasts or cubes of tofu (all protein). Or simply serve it hot with a mixture of rices and green beans or as an appetiser spread on small chunks of rye bread (carbohydrate).

100g (4oz) pitted black olives, chopped
2 tbsp capers, rinsed in milk to remove excess salt
2 cloves garlic, peeled and crushed
3 tbsp extra virgin olive or hazelnut oil
freshly ground black pepper
chopped fresh oregano, basil or thyme to taste

If using the tapenade to coat fish, chicken or tofu, pre-heat the oven to 180°C/350°F/gas mark 4.

Blend all the ingredients together in a food processor or pass them through a sieve to form a smooth paste. To coat the fish, chicken or tofu chunks, simply spread with the tapenade mixture and bake in the oven for 15–20 minutes.

Nut Butter FC (N)

Per 2 tsp serving:

Kcals	184.4
Fat	6.5g
Fibre	2.5g

Nut butter and chopped celery make an unusual and tasty filling for sandwiches and baked potatoes in their jackets. But nut butter is far more versatile than just a spread – try dabbing a little over cooked carrots, or adding a $1/2$ teaspoon to a salad dressing for extra flavour. (Cashew nuts have one of the lowest fat contents, but hazelnuts are fairly high in fat so use sparingly.)

450g (1lb) mixture of almonds, Brazil nuts, walnuts, hazelnuts or peanuts
$1/4$ tsp sea salt
4 tbsp (60ml) apple juice

Roast the nuts in a medium oven for 10–15 minutes, stirring occasionally. Grind to a fine paste in a coffee mill or food processor with a sharp blade. Dry roast the salt in a pan over a low heat for 1–2 minutes and add to the nut paste. Stir in just enough apple juice to make a thick purée. Store in screw-top jars. If the natural oil in the nuts separates, simply stir it back in. You can also make this recipe using seeds. For seeds such as sesame or sunflower seeds, dry roast in a pan over a low heat until the seeds crush easily when rubbed. Then proceed as before.

Raw Apple Sauce FC (N)

Serves 4

Per serving

Kcals	54
Fat	0.2g
Fibre	3.0g

Use this great tasting sauce to add spice to plain grilled pork chops, mackerel fillets or cold chicken.

4 eating apples, cored and chopped
juice of $1/2$ lemon
a pinch of grated nutmeg
a pinch of cinnamon
50–100ml (2–4fl oz) apple juice

Blend the apples with the lemon juice and spices in a food processor. Add sufficient apple juice to achieve a smooth consistency. The sauce may be warmed through gently in a saucepan if preferred, but do not let it boil.

DRESSINGS

Cucumber Dressing FC (P)

Per tbsp:

Kcals	6
Fat	0.02g
Fibre	0.1g

A creamy but refreshing dressing that also works well on baked potatoes and sliced avocados.

150g (5oz) cucumber
150g (5oz) natural low-fat, live yoghurt
1 tbsp olive oil
1 tbsp cider vinegar
1 sprig of dill
1/2 tsp dried dill seeds

Blend all the ingredients together in a food processor until the dressing is smooth and creamy. Store in the fridge.

Fine French Dressing FC (N)

Makes 300ml (1/2 pint) – stored in an air-tight jar in the fridge, this dressing will keep for up to a week. It is high in calories though, so use sparingly!

Per tsp:

Kcals	112
Fat	12g
Fibre	nil

175ml (6fl oz) sunflower oil or safflower oil
100ml (4fl oz) lemon juice
freshly ground black pepper
1/2 tsp mustard
1/4 tsp freshly grated root ginger
1–2 large cloves garlic, peeled and crushed

Put all the ingredients in a screw-top jar, replace the lid and shake vigorously to mix well. Store in the fridge.

Orange and Tamari Dressing FC (N)

Serves 12 as a salad dressing or 6 as a baked potato topping
Per tbsp:

Kcals	41
Fat	3.8g
Fibre	0.1g

This is very good with green-leafed vegetables such as raw spinach or salad leaves. It is also a useful dressing for those who don't like vinegar.

150ml (¹/₄ pint) freshly squeezed orange juice
1 tsp grated orange peel
2 tbsp tamari or soya sauce
1 tsp finely chopped fresh root ginger
3 tbsp olive oil
1 clove garlic, crushed

In a large bowl, mix all the ingredients together and stir well before using. Alternatively, place the ingredients into a large, screw-top jar, replace the lid and shake well. Store in the fridge.

Yoghurt and Chive Dressing FC (P)

Serves 6
Per tbsp:
Kcals   40
Fat   2.8g
Fibre   0.1g
150ml (¹/₄ pint) natural low-fat, live yoghurt
1 tbsp olive oil
1 tbsp lemon juice
1 tsp mustard
2 tbsp chopped chives
1 clove garlic, crushed
freshly ground black pepper, to season

In a large bowl, mix all the ingredients together, adding black pepper to season, and stir vigorously. Alternatively, place all the ingredients in a large, screw-top jar, replace the lid and shake well. Store in the fridge.

DESSERTS

Apricot Meringue

Serves 8
Per serving:
Kcals   131
Fat   9.3g
Fibre   4.2g

This deliciously light and fruity meringue recipe needs no added sugar as the apricots and bananas contain natural sugar – fructose – which is three times as sweet as processed sugar. It is the perfect dessert for a summer dinner party and can be kept in the fridge for up to two days if any is left over.

550g (1lb 4oz) apricots
75g (2oz) ground almonds
100g (4oz) peeled ripe banana

2 egg whites
50g (2oz) dessiccated coconut

Pre-heat the oven to 160°C/300°F/gas mark 2. Wash and roughly grate the apricots, add the ground almonds and pour into a 20cm (8") cake tin or baking dish. Blend the bananas in an electric blender, food processor or sieve so that they form a thick liquid. Whick the egg whites until they form stiff peaks and carefully fold into the liquid bananas. Then pour this topping evenly over the apricot and almond mixture and cook at the bottom of the oven for 30 minutes, until the surface just begins to brown in streaks. Remove the meringues from the oven and sprinkle the coconut on top before serving.

Bikini Diet Brownies

Makes 36 squares
Per serving:

Kcals	76
Fat	3.5g
Fibre	0.2g

This alternative fudge brownie recipe is remarkably low in calories so allows for that odd treat. It's made with prune purée instead of butter, so is much lower in fat. Because they are so rich, each serving is just 1" – so don't overeat!

100g (4oz) plain dark chocolate
150g (5oz) California prune purée
3 egg whites (size 2)
200g (7oz) soft light brown sugar
1 level tsp salt
1 tsp vanilla essence
65g (2¹/₂ oz) plain flour, sieved
25g (1oz) walnuts, chopped

Pre-heat the oven to 180°C/350°F/gas mark 4. Grease and line the bottom of a 15cm (6") square cake tin. Break the chocolate into a bowl and place over a saucepan of simmering water. Stir occasionally until the chocolate has melted. Remove from the heat and set aside to cool slightly. In a bowl mix together the prune purée, egg whites, sugar, salt and vanilla essence. Add the melted chocolate and stir until smooth. Fold in the sieved flour. Spread the mixture into the prepared tin, sprinkle with walnuts and bake for about 1 hour or until firm to the touch. Leave to cool completely. Cut into 36 2.5cm (1") squares.

Black Cherry Clafouti

Serves 4
Per serving:

Kcals	183
Fat	1.5g
Fibre	2.2g

To make the most of summer's seasonal harvest of black cherries, try baking them in this not-too-fattening version of a classic clafouti.

500g (17fl oz) fresh pitted cherries or jar-bottled black cherries, drained
dab of soft butter for greasing

Batter:
2 tbsp self-raising flour
2 tbsp caster sugar
1 pinch cinnamon
1 pinch fine salt
2 eggs
225ml (8fl oz) semi-skimmed milk
1 tbsp Kirsch or 1/2 tsp natural vanilla essence
1 tbsp icing sugar to serve
200ml (7fl oz) low-fat crème fraîche

Pre-heat the oven to 190°C/350°F/gas mark 5. Lightly grease a large shallow baking dish with soft butter and set aside.

To make the batter, sieve the flour into a mixing bowl, add the sugar, cinnamon and salt, then beat in the eggs to make a smooth battter. Gradually add the milk, and lastly the Kirsch or vanilla essence. Spread the cherries over the base of the baking dish, pour on the batter and bake in the centre of the oven for 40–45 minutes until brown at the edges. Allow to cool briefly, dredge with icing sugar and serve warm with low-fat crème fraîche.

Courgette and Carrot Cake FC (C)

Makes two 18cm (7") cakes
Per 4cm (1/2") wide slice:

Kcals	226
Fat	16.6g
Fibre	2.4g

This rich, dark cake tastes so delicious you won't believe it's so good for you! Less sweet than conventional recipes and healthier too! Butter is replaced with monounsaturated oil which also makes the mixture fabulously moist. I add coarsely chopped walnut pieces for extra crunch, but if baking for small children these should be finely ground to avoid the risk of choking. I find that dipping the spoon into hot water before spooning out the molasses and honey enables these sticky sweeteners to slide off the spoon more easily.

2 free-range eggs, size 3
2 tbsp crude blackstrap molasses
2 tbsp clear honey
150ml (1/4 pint) plus 1 tbsp walnut, hazelnut or olive oil
174g (6oz) buckwheat flour
1 tsp bicarbonate of soda
50g (2oz) natural wheatgerm

50g (2 oz) chopped walnuts
100g (4oz) carrots, scrubbed and grated
100g (4oz) courgettes, washed and grated
4 tbsp orange juice

Pre-heat the oven to 180°C/350°F/gas mark 4.

Lightly oil two Victoria sandwich tins. In a large mixing bowl, beat the eggs together before adding the molasses and honey. Stir vigorously before pouring in the oil. Fold in the buckwheat flour, bicarbonate of soda and wheatgerm, followed by the remaining ingredients. Pour into the baking tins and bake for 35–40 minutes, or until a metal skewer comes out clean. Allow to cool before turning out and slicing into wedges. Store in a tightly sealed container in a cool place.

Home-made Raspberry Yoghurt Ice FC (P)

Serves 6

Per serving:

Kcals	85
Fat	0.7g
Fibre	2.7g

Ice-cream is a minefield when it comes to avoiding sugar, saturated fat and artificial flavourings. Home-made yoghurt ice contains just three ingredients and is so easy to make, you'll wonder how you ever lived without it! This attractive dessert can also be made from strawberries and blackberries, or any other summer fruits.

275g (10oz) raspberries – fresh or frozen
50g (2oz) icing sugar
275ml (10fl oz) low-fat yoghurt
To serve:
350g (12oz) raspberries
6 sprigs mint
6 wafers (optional)

Adjust your freezer to its coldest setting, or have ready an ice-cream machine. Whizz the raspberries and sugar together in a food processor, transfer to a nylon sieve over a basin and rub the purée through with the back of a spoon. (If you don't mind raspberry seeds in your yoghurt ice, you can miss out this bit.) Combine the purée and yoghurt, then pour into a stainless steel or enamel bowl (plastic will slow the freezing process). Place the mixture in the freezer for one hour, then stir smoothly as it begins to freeze and return it to the freezer. Stir the yoghurt ice every 30 minutes until firm, (allow 3 hours). Home-made ices are best eaten once they become firm, as they have a tendency to harden if kept. Scoop the yoghurt ice into pretty glasses, scatter with fresh raspberries. Serve each with a wafer and a sprig of mint.

Mandarin Jelly FC (P)

Serves 4
Per serving:
Kcals   226
Fat   1.3g
Fibre   0.8g

This colourful jelly tastes great and my kids love it too. No artificial colourings or flavourings – just the pure goodness of fruit. Use freshly-squeezed orange juice if you can, or ruby orange juice to turn the jelly red. This dessert is an excellent source of vitamin C.

1 tin (300g) mandarins in natural juice
75fl oz (³/4 pint) orange juice
1 sachet or 3 tsp powdered gelatine

Drain the juice from the mandarins and mix with the orange juice. Place about half the liquid in a bowl and sprinkle in the gelatine. Heat gently until all the gelatine has dissolved. Add the remaining juice little by little, stirring continuously. Leave to cool for a couple of minutes, then sprinkle in the mandarins (they will sink to the bottom). Cover and chill in the fridge until set.

Mango Ice-Cream FC (P)

Serves 4
Per serving:
Kcals   103
Fat   0.4g
Fibre   4.3g

Make sure that the mangoes you use are really ripe and sweet to make a truly sumptuous low-fat ice-cream.

500g (1lb 2oz) ripe mango with the stone and skin removed
100ml (4fl oz) unsweetened apple juice
150g (5oz) low-fat fromage frais

Slice the mango and liquidise it in a blender with the apple juice and yoghurt to make a thick fruit purée. Chill the puréed fruit and if you have an ice-cream maker, pour it into the machine and follow the instructions given. Alternatively, you can use the freezer. Simply pour the fruit purée into a plastic container, cover and put in the freezer for about 45 minutes. Then remove from the freezer and whisk the mixture to get rid of any ice crystals that have formed. Return the container to the freezer and repeat the process after another 45 minutes. The ice-cream should then be firm and ready to serve or can be kept in the freezer until half an hour before you wish to serve it.

Plum Parfait

> *Serves 4*
> Per serving:
> Kcals   105
> Fat   0.4g
> Fibre   3.7g

Another perfect summer dessert, low in fat and sugar, with a deliciously spicy, fruity taste.

> *650g (1lb 7oz) plums*
> *150ml (5fl oz) unsweetened apple juice*
> *pinch cinnamon*
> *2 level tbsp cornflour*
> *1/2 tbsp brandy (optional)*
> *100ml (4fl oz) low-fat yoghurt*

Place half the plums in a heatproof bowl and cover with boiling water. After approximately 2 minutes, remove the plums from the water and peel away their skins. Then slice them and leave to one side. Purée the remainder of the plums with the apple juice in a blender and pour into a saucepan with the cinnamon and brandy. Remove a tablespoon of the liquid and mix with the cornflour before returning it to the pan. Then bring the mixture to the boil and simmer for a couple of minutes, stirring continuously as the purée thickens. Add the slices of plum to the pan and bring to the boil for about 15 seconds before transferring to a bowl. Allow the mixture to cool. To serve, you can attractively layer the fruit purée and yoghurt. First divide four-fifths of the fruit mixture into four bowls, put a tablespoon of yoghurt on top of the fruit, then cover with a tablespoon of the remaining fruit purée and finish with a large dot of yoghurt on top.

Rippled Fruit Fool FC (P)

> *Serves 4*
> Per serving:
> Kcals   127
> Fat   0.4g
> Fibre   7.0g

Fructose is a third sweeter than normal sugar so less is needed. I've used it in this delicious dessert, but you can use ordinary sugar instead.

> *450g (1lb) summer soft fruit, e.g. apricots, strawberries, raspberries*
> *2 large oranges, juice and grated rind*
> *40g (1 1/2 oz) fructose, fruit sugar (Fruisana or Dietade)*
> *125g (5oz) low-fat fromage frais or low-fat crème fraîche*
> *mint leaves to garnish*

In a medium saucepan dissolve the fruit sugar in the orange juice, add the chopped fruit and rind and cook briefly for one minute, stirring continuously just until the fruit begins to soften. Liquidise to a purée and pour into a bowl, stir in the fromage frais and gently fold in the fruit to give a rippled effect. Serve garnished with a little fresh fruit and mint leaves.

Spiced Bananas FC (C)

Serves 4
Per serving:
Kcals   198
Fat   10.5g
Fibre   1.1g

This recipe works well with pears too.

4 large ripe bananas
50g (2oz) butter
1 tbsp clear honey
2 tsp allspice

Peel and slice the bananas and place in four individual serving bowls. In a small saucepan quickly melt the butter and stir in the honey and allspice. Pour over the bananas and serve immediately. Another way to make this dish is to bake the fruit in a pre-heated oven at 180°C/350°F/gas mark 4 for 15 minutes to soften it, before pouring on the sauce and serving. Bake the bananas in their skins and they'll keep their colour better.

Strawberry Chinchilla with an Orange Sauce

Serves 4
Per serving:
Kcals   199
Fat   0.4g
Fibre   2.3g

This beautifully light soufflé dessert is made with half the amount of sugar used to make conventional meringue and is decked with strawberries.

dab of soft butter or margarine for greasing
4 egg whites
100g (4oz) caster sugar
Orange sauce:
225ml (8fl oz) water
2 tbsp caster sugar
2 tbsp cornflour
2 tbsp frozen orange concentrate
450g (1lb) strawberries, hulled and halved if large

Pre-heat the oven to 180°C/350°F/gas mark 4. Bring a kettle of water to the boil. Apply a scant layer of soft butter to the inside of a 2-pint soufflé dish and stand in a deep roasting tray. Whisk the egg white in a clean bowl until soft but not grainy. Gradually add the sugar and whisk until smooth. Turn the meringue into the soufflé dish. Half fill the roasting tray with boiling water and bake near the bottom of the oven for 25 minutes. To make the orange sauce, measure the water and sugar into a small saucepan and simmer to dissolve the sugar. Put the cornflour into a cup, combine with a tablespoon of cold water. Stir the cornflour into the syrup and simmer to thicken. Allow to cool, then stir in the orange juice concentrate. When the chinchilla is cooked, remove from the oven and allow to settle for 5 minutes before turning out on to a serving plate. Top the chinchilla with as many strawberries as you can and serve at room temperature with orange sauce and extra strawberries. Strawberry chinchilla can be made 3–4 hours in advance.

Strawberry Sorbet FC (N)

Serves 6
Per serving:

Kcals	24
Fat	0.1g
Fibre	0.7g

This healthy dessert is an excellent source of the nutrients vitamin C and beta-carotene, so you can eat it with a clear conscience.

450g (1lb) fresh strawberries
juice of 1 large orange

Blend the ingredients together in a food processor until smooth. Pour into a bowl or container and place in the freezer for 1 hour. Remove and allow the mixture to thaw slightly, if necessary, then beat well with a metal spoon to break up any ice crystals and return the sorbet to the freezer for at least 5 hours. Allow to soften at room temperature for 15 minutes before serving.

Summer Strawberries in a Raspberry and Passion-fruit Sauce FC (N)

Serves 4
Per serving:

Kcals	134
Fat	0.6g
Fibre	9.6g

350g (12oz) fresh or frozen raspberries
3 tbsp caster sugar
1 passion-fruit
750g (1lb 8oz) strawberries, hulled and halved if large
4 sponge fingers (optional) **(C)**

Put the raspberries and sugar in a small saucepan, and soften over a low heat to release the juices. Simmer for 5 minutes, allow to cool. Turn the raspberries into a food processor. Halve the passion-fruit, scoop out the seeds and juices, add to the raspberries and blend smoothly. Pass the fruit sauce through a nylon sieve positioned over a bowl to remove the seeds and pips. Fold the strawberries into the sauce and serve at room temperature with sponge fingers, if desired. This will make it a carbohydrate dessert.

Section 6

THE BODY BEAUTIFUL

BEATING CELLULITE

Losing weight is not the only consideration if you want to look good in that bikini! Cellulite on the hips and thighs can give even the thinnest thighs an unattractive, dimpled appearance. This dreaded orange-peel effect seems to afflict the majority of women at some point during their lives and it is notoriously hard to shift. Anticellulite creams and lotions are big business and anyone who can come up with an overnight solution to cellulite will become an instant millionaire.

Cellulite is frequently dismissed by sceptics, usually male, as being no different from ordinary fat. This can easily be challenged by looking around you as slim women also have cellulite; although it does tend to be more obvious on those who are overweight. Likewise, being overweight does not mean that you will automatically develop lumpy cellulite deposits. The link between cellulite and fat is simply this; cellulite arises among the fat cells in the layer of fatty tissue beneath the skin, especially on the upper legs and buttocks, where women tend to store their reserves of fat. Another popular area for cellulite is above the knees and on the upper arms where we tend to store any excess fat. Cellulite is the name given to toxins which are stored in fatty deposits well away from the body's vital organs. Those nasty lumps and bumps are an indication that there is an unhealthy build-up of toxins which the body is unable to get rid of.

THE APPEARANCE OF CELLULITE

In its mildest form, cellulite looks a bit like orange peel, creating slight ripples in the skin's surface, but when severe, the bumps beneath the skin are much larger and more obvious. If you are not sure whether you have cellulite, a good way of testing your skin is to pinch a small area of your thigh between two fingers and, if you have cellulite, the texture will be granular and lumpy, very much like cottage cheese. Don't worry if you do discover that you have cellulite – it can be significantly improved and even banished entirely by a combination of a change in diet, skin brushing, massage and exercise.

DUMPING GROUND

Under a microscope, cellulite tissue reveals fat cells which are saturated with fluid and wastes which are trapped in a fine network of hardened connective fibres. These wastes are toxic substances which our bodies are unable to make use of. According to holistic GP Richard James, one of the properties of fat deposits is to absorb poisonous substances which the body cannot deal with, preventing the poisons from harming our vital organs. Our fat deposits lock these poisons away indefinitely so that those who have had cellulite for ten years or more are probably storing toxins that are ten years' old! This is one reason why cellulite is so hard to shift. Dr James claims that all fat-soluble substances, including herbicides and pesticides, are naturally attracted to fatty tissue which explains why the toxins in women make a bee-line for the hips and thighs. The walls of our fat cells are surrounded by extra deposits of collagen and they soon develop into porridge-like structures called 'micronodules'. These may later join together to form larger 'macronodules' which cause the dreaded dimpled appearance under the skin's surface.

THE ONSET OF CELLULITE

What causes cellulite? There are many answers to this million-dollar question. Poor circulation is mainly to blame as blood is a rich source of oxygen and nutrients which our cells need in order to function properly. If we bombard our bodies with toxic substances, such as alcohol and chemically treated processed food, a build-up of toxins will occur which interferes with our circulation and absorption of these vital nutrients. An inadequate flow of blood to the capillaries which serve the fat cells means short rations of oxygen and nutrients, and only a partial removal of toxins via the lymphatic system. Lymph is a fluid that flows around the body through a vast network of vessels. Lymph vessels contain a huge amount of white blood cells which attack invaders and clean out waste, but these can become easily clogged by a diet which is too rich in red meat, dairy products, sugar, fried and processed food, all of which the body finds more difficult to digest and metabolise.

When these 'bad' foods are only partially digested, there is a build-up of waste which ferments inside us and soon becomes toxic. On top of the toxins in our diet, the impurities in our water and in the air that we breathe all add up to a considerable amount of waste. Fortunately, our bodies are equipped with a safety device that locks these toxins away in our fat cells well away from our vital organs. Our organs of detoxification play a very important part in getting rid of waste and if one of these organs is not doing its job properly, then extra pressure is put on the other organs of detoxification; for example, constipation, which can often go unrecognised, adds enormously to the body's rubbish load as it traps waste matter inside us.

This waste material is stored throughout the body in organs, tissues, cells and in spaces in between cells, known as interstitial spaces. These areas contain a fluid, lymph, which has the double role of feeding our cells with vital nutrients and carrying away any waste matter. The fatty tissue on the thighs, where circulation is sluggish, is particularly prone to collecting waste because the exchange of waste for nutrients is less effective here. These cells soon become congested, taking its toll on the capillaries and causing their fragile walls to weaken. This eventually causes a serious build-up of fluid, which pushes cells and capillaries further apart and undermines the body's waste disposal system. As a result, there is an accumulation of fat, toxins and fluids which are, in effect, bundles of cellulite in its early stages. These bundles move upwards into the middle layer of our skin, where the fat cells clump together to form nodules. These nodules expand and become trapped in fibrous tissue, compressing our blood capillaries and causing even further congestion. And so cellulite is born.

THE LYMPHATIC SYSTEM

To understand how to banish cellulite and prevent its return we need to take a closer look at how our bodies get rid of waste. The main waste disposal system is the lymphatic drainage system. The tiny capillaries, or lymphatics, in the subcutaneous tissue beneath our skin drain the liquid waste from the spaces between our cells and transport it through strategically placed lymph nodes towards the lymphatic ducts in the upper body. This liquid is known as lymph and it is filtered by the lymphatic ducts before returning through the heart into the bloodstream, where it is further processed by the eliminative organs, such as the kidneys and liver.

Unfortunately, the lymphatic system does not automatically run smoothly, as research carried out at the Université Libre in Brussels has clearly shown. Tests on women suffering from cellulite revealed that 100 percent were affected by poor lymphatic drainage. The difference between blood and lymphatic circulation is that the lymph does not have a powerful pump like the heart to drive it. The movement of the lymph towards the heart depends partly on the compression of lymphatic vessels by the muscles in our limbs, and partly on the 'suction' created by the movements of respiration, so the way in which we breathe is very important – long deep breaths are best.

In addition, the lymph often has a long way to travel before it is filtered by one of the lymphatic ducts. The right lymphatic duct, which is located just inside the right collarbone, is only required to filter the lymph from the upper right-hand side of the body, but the poor old thoracic duct in the chest has to drain lymph from the left side of the head, neck and chest, the left arm and the entire body below the ribs – a massive job! This may explain why almost everyone has more cellulite on their right leg than their left because the waste from that region has to take a long, circular route to the relevant filtering station without the benefit of a forceful mechanism, like the heart, to help it on its way.

THE GENDER ISSUE

Why is it that women are the only victims of cellulite? It does seem grossly unfair – but the reason is actually a good one. It is not that men are immune to the dangers of excess weight and internal pollution, it is just that they deal with it in a different way. For one thing, men store their fat in a different place – usually around the midriff and closer to the vital organs. Although they are rarely troubled by the 'orange-peel' phenomenon in this area, they do suffer from a relatively higher incidence of heart disease up to middle age. Women, up to middle age, experience a great deal of hormonal activity due to menstruation and pregnancy and these hormonal imbalances, in particular high levels of oestrogen, are often to blame for the development of cellulite. In simple terms, high levels of oestrogen encourage our bodies to store toxins in the fatty tissue in our thighs and buttocks well away from our vital organs. This is excellent for our health, but not so great if we want to look good in a bikini...

FEMALE HORMONES

So women's bodies are programmed to function differently to men's and this is primarily due to hormones. Few of us realise just how important hormones are. They are responsible for our libido, our moods, the appearance of our skin and, of course, for reproduction. It is the female sex hormones which are responsible for the development of breasts, underarm and pubic hair and the typically feminine proportions of the body. These include the fat deposits which start to appear on the hips, thighs and shoulders from puberty onwards. Oestrogen and progesterone are the main players and they regulate the menstrual cycle and maintain pregnancy, or prevent it when hormones are taken in a synthetic form – the contraceptive pill. These powerful hormones also interact with another hormone, aldosterone (shared by both sexes), to control fluid balance.

WATER RETENTION

Over the last sixty years or so, French research has revealed a number of important facts about the nature of cellulite. It has been discovered that water retention is at the heart of the problem and oestrogen encourages women to retain fluid. Whenever there is a burst of sex hormones, the body is programmed to store fat for later use – in pregnancy or for breastfeeding. But the poor circulation which is associated with fatty tissues means that the area becomes a bit of dead end where fluids which cannot be released build up. Excessive levels of oestrogen are a powerful trigger for the onset of cellulite and may be the principal cause in a staggering 75 percent of cases. 12 percent are believed to coincide with puberty, when the ovaries become active and oestrogen production starts; 17 percent with pregnancy, which demands an increased supply of oestrogen and progesterone and can be accompanied by extra weight-gain and poor circulation; and 27 percent of cases in the run-up to the menopause, when progesterone production falls, again sending oestrogen levels out of balance. A further 19 percent of cellulite conditions are linked to oral contraceptives which also encourage water retention and weight-gain. This explains why many women on the pill who eat healthily and regularly exercise, nevertheless find it impossible to shift cellulite no matter what lengths they go to.

WHY ME?

Some women are fortunate enough never to develop cellulite regardless of how high their hormone levels rise. This is due to a number of different factors, some of which may be hereditary, such as body shape, and other factors include the activity of the lymphatic drainage system and diet. Dr Terence Ryan, consultant dermatologist and clinical professor of dermatology at the Churchill Hospital in Headington, Oxford, observes that the female tendency to develop cellulite is strongly linked to anatomical type and that so called 'pear-shaped' women are particularly prone to developing cellulite. Women with slow metabolisms, who put on weight easily and lose it with difficulty, are also especially prone. There are other anatomical features which tip the balance against women. They have twice the amount of fatty tissue as men, which, given the principal part played by the fat in the cellulite saga, does stack the odds against them. Women also have less collagen in their skin than men and this makes cellulite more obvious. In addition, the skin tissue on female thighs is more loosely structured and, therefore, more easily disrupted by the toxin and fluid build-up responsible for the formation of cellulite.

HOW TO COMBAT CELLULITE

If hormonal imbalance is the cause of your cellulite, it will be difficult to banish it entirely unless your hormones become stable again. However, you should be able to improve the appearance of your skin significantly by adopting a four-pronged approach to cellulite which involves diet, exercise, skin brushing and massage. Alternatively, if you think that the contraceptive pill is the cause of your cellulite, then you may wish to consider using some other form of contraception in order to shed any excess weight and those unattractive lumps and bumps. It is generally a good idea to take the odd break from the contraceptive pill as it affects our bodies in many ways, which the development of cellulite clearly demonstrates. You may decide to stop taking the contraceptive pill a couple of months before the summer; so that your hormone levels have a chance to return to normal and hopefully any excess weight and cellulite will banish in time for your summer holiday. However, it is important to remember that although your menstruation cycle will be irregular after taking the pill, you must ensure that you are using some other form of contraception during your break from it unless you want to become pregnant.

The anticellulite plan

If the cause of your cellulite does not seem to be purely hormonal, such as the contraceptive pill, then adopting this anticellulite plan will help you to get rid of cellulite so that you can reveal a smooth-skinned body in your bikini. This approach to combating cellulite is the only one that really works as, for many of us, the cellulite has built up over a number of years and the toxins are locked in our fatty deposits and have no desire to move. To remove cellulite effectively we need to adopt the following strategy:

* a low-fat diet which is rich in fresh fruit and vegetables
* skin brushing
* lymphatic drainage massage
* exercise (see page 160).

THE BIKINI DIET FOR A CELLULITE-FREE BODY

Sadly, the 'modern' diet – a far cry from the natural wholefood diet of our ancestors – is a minefield for the cellulite sufferer because of its high sugar and fat content and emphasis on refined and processed foods instead of the wealth of fresh, natural ingredients that are available to us. The human body is polluted by this diet as there is only so much rubbish that our liver, kidneys and bowel are able to process and eliminate. Once they have reached their capacity, the only alternative is for those substances to remain in the system. What we take into our bodies affects our general well-being and the healthy state of all our tissues – including the skin. It is also of critical importance if you are trying to get rid of cellulite and prevent it from recurring in the future. The *Bikini Diet* is a low-fat diet full of fresh ingredients which are rich in the nutrients our bodies require to flush out toxins and build strong, healthy, and above all smooth, skin.

Toxic stimulants

In addition to following the *Bikini Diet*, you will also need to steer clear of toxins wherever possible if you are serious about combating cellulite. This means cutting down on, or entirely avoiding, toxic stimulants such as alcohol, caffeine and nicotine as these all enable cellulite to flourish. Alcohol, especially spirits, is a very concentrated source of fuel as well as being a poison to the body. When consumed in excess, it ends up as surplus to requirements and is added to the fat stores. If you drink wine, you may also be consuming an unhealthy dose of colourings, flavourings and pesticides, unless it is organically produced. The toxic effect of alcohol rapidly penetrates our bodies. When we take a sip of alcohol, it immediately enters the bloodstream through the intestine and is then swiftly transported to our cells. Tolerance varies from one individual to the next, but it is far lower in women than men. The adverse effects of alcohol have a considerable bearing on cellulite formation, depleting stores of essential fats and vitamin C which are essential for healthy skin. Alcohol also puts extra strain on the liver, a particularly vital organ of detoxification, and interferes with cell-to-cell communication which again hampers the disposal of waste. With our extensive knowledge of the many dangers of smoking and the sobering fact that smokers dramatically reduce their life expectancy with the threat of lung, throat and mouth cancers and coronary heart disease, you would think that we should be a nation that did not smoke. Sadly, this is not the case and many continue to smoke regardless of the fact that they are distributing carcinogenic substances into the atmosphere, as well as into themselves. When smoking tobacco, numerous toxins are inhaled into the body where they not only overload our organs of detoxification, they also contribute to serious disease processes. In addition, these toxins deplete our bodies of the nutrients, such as vitamin C, which we need to form healthy tissues. This is why smokers tend to have older-looking skin with more premature lines than the rest of us.

Fat in food

Fatty foods are also cellulite-forming foods. Fat is difficult to digest and it leaves behind a residue which interferes with the digestion of the foods that follow. This has a cumulative effect of wastes getting trapped in the intestine, causing toxins to be reabsorbed into the blood, while the fatty coating on the intestine walls makes the channel even narrower, blocking the absorption of nutrients. Even the lymph, which plays a key role in reducing cellulite, takes on the viscous quality of fatty substances and this interferes further with the elimination of waste.

Sugar and salt

The food scientists and marketing wizards are only too aware of the addictive qualities of both of these staple additives which they use without restraint to get our taste-buds hooked. You only have to read the labels on the packets to see this. The level of salt (or sodium) in the body has an important role to play in regulating fluids. Sodium works with the mineral potassium to balance the fluid content, and an excess of salt threatens the all-important sodium–potassium balance both inside and outside the cells, encouraging fluid retention in our tissues. This waterlogging, always intensified around the hips and thighs, creates the perfect conditions for tissue congestion to occur, and for cellulite to flourish.

Junk

The last word must be reserved for 'junk' food as it has a lot to answer for. The advent of 'junk' or processed or convenience food, call it what you will, which has invaded our high streets and supermarket shelves has seriously affected our overall health. While the huge list of additives and preservatives may produce a successful product that keeps us coming back for more, it dramatically reduces the majority of the nutrients which were present in the food originally. In other words, nutritionally speaking, the food is a pale shadow of its former self.

More importantly, we are now taking in a larger quantity and variety of chemical substances which our body has not evolved a way of dealing with. In addition to the chemicals showered over fruit and vegetables, most of our meat is contaminated by residues of steroids, hormones and antibiotics which are fed to livestock. Our bodies are unable to process these chemicals and so we store them instead. Inevitably, some of them end up in the poor old thighs causing absolute havoc, and no doubt leaving a trail of destruction behind them as they pass through the system. Dr Elisabeth Dancey who specialises in mesotherapy at her clinic in Wimpole Street, London, treating cellulite amongst other conditions sums up the problem: 'Not all of us can metabolise artificial substances. We don't have the enzyme systems to deal with them, so they just hang around, damaging tissue like a spanner in the works.'

SKIN BRUSHING

This activity was previously frowned upon as only for masochists, but now most health practitioners see it as something very beneficial. More importantly, it is essential if you want to improve the texture of your skin and banish cellulite forever as it stimulates both your circulation and your lymphatic drainage system. A brush made from natural fibres on a wooden base is ideal, and a long detachable handle is required to get to those hard-to-reach areas of the back. These wooden brushes are relatively cheap and are available from most chemists.

Daily skin brushing removes the dead skin from our pores, allowing them to breathe and absorb any anticellulite creams and essential oils which we may wish to apply afterwards. Furthermore, it leaves the pores unblocked so that the skin can eliminate toxins effectively through them. The skin is the largest eliminative organ, and if it cannot function properly, enormous pressure is put on the other eliminative organs in the body such as the bowels, lungs and kidneys. Few of us are aware of the extent to which our pores are blocked by dead skin cells, sebum, sweat, bacteria and pollutants. A quick wash with soap and water may not unblock clogged pores – your skin needs to be brushed with a coarse, bristle brush. Try brushing your skin in direct sunlight and you will see hundreds of tiny flakes of dead skin fly away from your body.

Body brushing also stimulates blood flow and carries oxygen to where the body needs it. It involves long, relatively hard brush strokes towards the heart and this greatly stimulates circulation and the lymphatic drainage system. Try to brush your body every day for a couple of weeks and then limit it to a couple of days a week, varying the days, so as to 'surprise' your skin and maintain the beneficial effects of skin brushing. It may seem hard and uncomfortable at first, but your body will soon get used to this new feeling and you can then use firmer brush strokes. Most people grow to enjoy the tingling sensation derived from body brushing and feel that it is as much a part of their daily routine as brushing their teeth. In any case, it is an excellent way to start the day, as the blood starts to course through your veins supplying every inch of your body with the energy-giving nutrients that it requires. You are left feeling revitalised and ready for action!

How to skin-brush

It is best to brush your skin before a bath or shower as this will dislodge dirt and dead skin which can then be washed away leaving your pores completely clean and ready to absorb any anticellulite creams and oils which you apply after washing. You should start to brush from your extremities, i.e. your hands and feet, up towards your heart. Starting at your fingertips, brush in long, firm strokes along the palms and backs of your hands up towards your elbows and shoulders. Then do your feet, brushing over the soles, across the toes, round the

Always brush your body using long, firm strokes in the direction of the heart.

ankles and up to the knees. Brush over the backs of the knees and then home in on the main cellulite zone, the upper leg, to dislodge those nasty lumpy bits. You may want to take a little longer over this area and vary your upward strokes to include some circular movements over the outer thighs and buttocks and in towards the inner thighs where the lymph nodes are located. A gentle clockwise motion is ideal over the abdomen. Do not forget to brush up the sides of your body and the lower back, where toxins can easily collect. Stop once you are level with the heart and then brush downwards from the upper part of your body, over the neck and shoulders. Finally, rotate the brush gently on the inner side of your armpits towards your breast where more lymph nodes are located. (See the diagram opposite.)

A word of warning: Avoid broken, inflamed or infected skin. If you suffer from eczema or psoriasis or have any varicose veins, do not brush near affected areas. If you find the brush too rough, it is a good idea to soak it in warm water then allow it to dry naturally overnight. In any case, you will need to wash it every few weeks for hygienic reasons. The odours that your brush will take up in the first few weeks are proof that something is being eliminated!

LYMPHATIC DRAINAGE MASSAGE

Massage is another valuable weapon in the battle against cellulite, which supports your efforts on the diet and exercise front. Like skin brushing, it can speed up the general cleansing process by activating the return of blood to the heart and the lymph to the lymphatic ducts. Frequent massage of problem areas over a period of time can also whittle away stubborn deposits of cellulite. Lymphatic drainage massage with detoxifying essential oils is particularly effective in combating cellulite, especially when carried out by a professional, as the lymphatic system plays such an important part in controlling the toxic build-up in cells and tissues. Lymph flows through tiny channels that lead to lymph nodes, where the lymph is cleansed before it is filtered and released into the bloodstream via ducts. The more toxic you are and the less exercise you have, the more sluggish your lymphatic drainage system will be.

To stimulate the lymphatic drainage system through massage, you need to apply gentle pressure to the body using your fingers which should move slowly up the body in the direction of the lymph (see the diagram). If the massage is too vigorous, it will overload the system and may also cause broken blood vessels and bruising. Particular attention should be paid to the lymph glands which are situated in the neck, armpits, backs of the knees and the groin. Begin massaging the hands and arms up to your shoulders. Use small, gentle movements, paying particular attention to the lymph glands in your armpits. Then massage each leg up to the groin. The back of each thigh should also be massaged many times into the groin area. The direction of the massage on the lower back should be outwards from the spine to each side of the body, and on your lower front you need to massage downwards towards your groin. The massage on the upper part of your body (front and back), should be directed towards the nearest armpit. Finally, the back of the neck should be massaged outwards from the centre and down the front to the base of the neck where two more lymph nodes are situated.

The black dots represent the lymph nodes, while the arrows represent the direction in which the lymph flows. Massage along these lines in slow movements to stimulate the lymphatic drainage system.

ADDITIONAL HELP

Essential oils

The essential oils extracted from plants contain a wealth of active ingredients, which, when absorbed by the skin, help to eliminate toxins and reduce cellulite. Some of these ingredients strengthen our blood vessels and boost circulation, while others drain the waterlogged tissue and reduce inflammation. Certain essential oils can help to balance our hormones while others tone and soften the skin and all these actions can play a part in reducing cellulite. Essential oils can be added to your bath water where they are absorbed by the skin. Alternatively you can add a few drops of an essential oil to a carrier oil, such as grapeseed or almond oil, and massage a little into your skin after washing. It is important to obtain your oils from a reliable source, since their effectiveness rests on the quality of raw materials and the extraction methods used. Essential oils are costly because so little is extracted from each plant, but a little goes a long way.

Different oils possess different qualities and there are a number of aromatic essences specifically recommended for the treatment of cellulite. These include basil, celery, Atlas cedarwood, cypress, sweet fennel, grapefruit, juniper, lavender, patchouli and rosemary.

Anticellulite baths

Add these essential oils to your bath water just before you get in to enjoy a fifteen-minute soak:

(a) 4 drops geranium + 4 drops rosemary
(b) 4 drops sweet fennel + 4 drops juniper
(c) 4 drops basil + 4 drops lavender
(d) 4 drops patchouli + 4 drops mandarin

Anticellulite massage oils

Follow your aromatic bath with one of the following:
To 100ml (4fl oz) grapeseed oil add either:
(a) 10 drops juniper + 5 drops mandarin + 5 drops sweet fennel
(b) 8 drops geranium + 6 drops rosemary + 6 drops basil

Detox herbs and supplements

There are a number of natural foods that are difficult to incorporate into our daily diet which are highly effective at detoxifying our systems and banishing cellulite. These can be taken instead in supplement form and they include sea vegetables – different forms of algae – which, believe it or not, are highly nutritious and promote digestion and metabolism of food.

All seaweeds are rich in the minerals which our bodies need in order for their metabolic processes to function properly. Some of these minerals are only needed by the body in minute amounts but, because our normal food sources have been depleted of much of their nutritional value due to modern farming methods and pollution, we need to get certain nutrients elsewhere. Some sea plants are rich in special forms of fibre called alginates which have the ability to bind with toxins in the body and remove them. They are also rich in organic iodine which tends to stimulate metabolic processes. Kelp can be bought in supplement form, but make sure that it has been collected from unpolluted waters and then 'atomised', or broken into very fine particles. This process of atomisation is very important because seaweeds tend to have very hard cell walls and these walls need to be broken down to allow our bodies access to their mineral content.

Cleansing herbs

Many herbs have a cleansing effect on the body which will help to boost this anticellulite programme. They can be drunk in the form of herbal teas or added fresh to salads and other meals. Some herbs are natural diuretics which means that they provoke an increase in the flow of urine and this is one way to rid the body of toxins and put a stop to water retention. Dandelion leaves, parsley, celery, asparagus, horsetail and juniper are particularly good herbal diuretics. Other herbs help to eliminate wastes through the skin by encouraging perspiration, such as ginger and peppermint. Formulations of many detoxifying herbs are available in pill or capsule form, but it is better to eat the natural plants, where available. One of the herbs which we do not get from our diet is ginkgo biloba. The leaves of the ginkgo biloba tree are highly antioxidant, so prevent cell damage, and their bioflavonoid content helps to protect our capillary walls. Ginkgo biloba extract is available in tablet form and it helps to boost circulation, which is also good news for the skin. It is also currently being investigated for use in anticellulite creams.

Anticellulite products

In addition to the efforts you make with your diet, your exercise plan and your bathing routines, there is a whole world of products out there boasting about their cellulite-reducing powers. However, anticellulite creams, lotions, gels and oils, are very unlikely to have any more than a light toning or firming effect on the skin unless they are backed up by dietary changes and increased physical activity. Massage is usually recommended once the cream has been applied, as it encourages the ingredients to penetrate the deeper layers of skin. The majority of anticellulite creams contain natural herbs which are renowned for their detoxifying properties, such as butcher's broom, horsetail and ivy. One of the most recent developments in anticellulite creams is the use of the drug aminophylline. This drug was originally used to treat asthma patients until scientists at the Stanford University in California discovered that it breaks down fat and disperses it away from the legs and thighs. Although the content of this drug in creams is usually very low (2 percent), some women have developed a rash from using the creams.

Stress and exercise

Stress, lack of sleep and not enough exercise also contribute to the formation of deposits. When we become stressed, our hypothalamus gland is stimulated and it releases the hormone adrenaline and increases our blood sugar level to deal with the emergency. This high blood sugar is not needed, so it gets laid down on the thighs as fat. The hypothalamus gland also inhibits certain processes during stress causing water retention and high blood pressure. Prolonged stress can also disrupt normal eating patterns, induce sugar cravings and interfere with digestion, elimination and breathing. So, if you feel yourself becoming stressed, take deep breaths and try to relax by thinking about something pleasant.

Regular exercise is also needed to stimulate the removal of cellulite and create a smooth, slim body. Sitting or standing in one position for extended periods of time during your working and leisure hours will, inevitably, result in slower circulation and an underactive metabolism. By encouraging deeper breathing and stimulating sluggish circulation and lymphatic drainage, exercise can actually help with the removal of excess fluid and toxins which accumulate in the spaces between our cells. It also speeds up the rate at which we burn fat, even when we are not exercising. See Exercise Extras on page 160.

Body scrubs

Other methods for improving the skin's texture and tone include body scrubs. These are best carried out either before or during a shower, as they tend to be quite messy. Body scrubs involve massaging the skin with a gritty substance to shift dead skin cells and embedded grime, and improve the appearance of spots and pimples. Let's face it – none of us like to reveal a back covered with pimples! Getting rid of all our dead skin will also give us a smoother tan.

Body scrubs can either be used on their own or in conjunction with a rough flannel or loofah to increase their effectiveness. Loofahs themselves are the long, fibrous pod of the *Luffa aegyptiaca* plant, which has been used as a body scrubber since ancient Egyptian times. Massage pads and mitts can be made from pieces of loofah and these are good for scrubbing smaller areas of skin such as the hands and the soles of the feet. Loofahs should be kept clean by rinsing them in clean water after each use and hung up to dry to prevent them from becoming mouldy.

Peanut butter scrub

This body scrub is rich in natural oils that leave the skin feeling soft and smooth.

50g (2oz) crunchy peanut butter
25g (1oz) finely ground sea salt
30ml (2tbsp) almond oil

Mix together the peanut butter and the sea salt and stir in the almond oil. The mixture should form a soft paste. Rub on to damp skin, all over the body, concentrating on areas of hard skin on the elbows, upper arms and knees. Rinse off with warm water and shower as usual.

Bust scrub

Most skin scrubs are too abrasive to use on the delicate skin that covers the breasts, but a gentle skin scrub is a good way to preserve skin tone and to remove any flakiness from the breasts or nipple area.

25g (1oz) medium ground oatmeal
25g (1oz) finely ground almonds
15ml (1tbsp) almond oil

Mix together the oatmeal and the almonds with the almond oil to form a paste. Apply to dampened skin and massage into the neck and chest area with firm but gentle circular movements. Always massage upwards to avoid pulling the skin and encouraging slackening. Rinse thoroughly and shower as usual. You will find the skin is left feeling especially soft and smooth.

Hip and thigh scrub

This is my favourite body treatment as it is very simple to do and really works wonders on the skin. It is ideal for shifting patches of stubborn cellulite and should be carried out at least twice a week to see the best results.

30ml (2tbsp) grapeseed oil
5 drops juniper essential oil
2 drops lemon essential oil
75g (3oz) polenta or cornmeal

In a screw-top bottle or jar, mix together the grapeseed oil with the essential oils and shake well. Pour the oil mixture over the cornmeal and mix to form a gritty paste. Apply to dampened skin on the hips, buttocks and thighs. Massage firmly, using sweeping, circular movements in an upwards direction. (For greater effect, use a rough flannel or massage mitt instead of the hands.) Massage for at least two minutes before rinsing the gritty particles away. Any mixture left over can be rubbed into the feet, hands and upper arms to leave them exceptionally smooth and glowing.

ANTICELLULITE TACTICS

Before you embark on this anticellulite regime it is important to tell yourself that you can beat cellulite and achieve the results you want. Think forward to the time when you can feel proud of your body and at ease in whatever clothes you wish to wear, including that stunning bikini. You may have a wardrobe full of clothes which are a little longer, fuller and maybe darker than you would choose, but which have done a good job in camouflaging a bottom-heavy silhouette. Perhaps you have even written off clothes that you are convinced you have 'outgrown'. Be prepared for a pleasant surprise – but be realistic. You cannot change your body type or the size of your bones. However, there is a lot you can do to remodel the flesh that clothes it and undo the damage which has caused it to sag, dimple and bulge.

The bottom line

As the weeks progress, you will be able to watch as the lines of your body are resculptured and the lumps and bumps, which you had begun to assume were here to stay, gradually disappear. Needless to say, these sort of changes do not occur overnight, nor will they happen without a great deal of effort on your part, but I am sure that you will agree that the smooth, slim silhouette that will emerge makes it all worthwhile. We have seen that the causes of cellulite are numerous, and the build-up cumulative. Hormones, stress, poor diet and bad habits will all have played their part over the years, or decades, gradually adding to the cellulite burden. Time and an all-encompassing approach are what are now required to undo the damage.

This may mean a radical rethink of your diet, your exercise routine (or lack of it) and a new strategy to deal with the pressures in your life. If you stand back, you may be able to see the factors of your lifestyle which have contributed to the problem, such as smoking. It is up to you to reverse these trends and adopt a fresh approach which will tackle the problem from both the outside and from within. Your immediate aim is to spring-clean your overburdened system, while setting your sights on the longer-term goal of limiting the build-up of toxins in the future. It may seem like an enormous task, but the rewards are huge and extend far beyond reclaiming your smooth, cellulite-free body. You will find yourself with greater stores of energy and self-confidence.

BEATING ACNE

It is all very well having smooth, cellulite-free skin, but if you have a spotty back it is not going to look good in a bikini or backless swimsuit. If your skin is covered in acne it is important to keep it as clean as possible and skin brushing, body scrubs and mud packs will all help to get rid of dead skin and grime which block the pores and aggravates acne.

CONCEALERS

If you have any body scars, broken blood vessels or spots which you do not want to show to the world, then Dermablend have an extensive range of water-proof body make-up which is ideal for covering up these blemishes. Their Leg and Body Cover is available in ten different colours from the palest skin to black and it lasts all day (see Useful Addresses).

HAIR REMOVAL

Another consideration before hitting the beach is excess body hair, normally hidden from view but exposed in all its glory during the summer. Hairy legs and underarms and pubic hair poking out from the sides of a bikini are not attractive. Body hair is perceived as unfeminine and anti-erotic and western women have taken pains to remove it throughout history. In 3000 BC the ancient Egyptians rubbed themselves with dried papyrus leaves to remove all body hair. Later the ancient Greeks and Romans removed all body hair using razors, tweezers and pumice stones. Fortunately, today there are a hundred and one different methods of removing hair – the most popular methods are listed here.

BLEACHING

Instead of removing the soft hairs on your face or forearms and taking the risk that the hairs will grow back coarser, it is a good idea to bleach the hairs so that they are less obvious. It is a totally painless process and root colour tends to come in very slowly so that it does not have to be repeated too often. If you spend a lot time in the sun, your hairs will eventually be bleached naturally by the sun's rays. Many women are allergic to bleaching products so test them on a small patch of your skin, such as the inner elbow, first.

DEPILATORY CREAMS

Depilatory creams and mousses are used by many women to remove all kinds of body hair, especially from around the bikini line. These work by dissolving the hair below the skin's surface and it takes a week or so for the hair to grow back. Unfortunately, these creams contain strong chemicals and often have a pungent smell. They also take five to ten minutes to work. However, depilatory creams are a longer-lasting method of hair removal than shaving and are ideal for the bikini area.

ELECTROLYSIS

This is an expensive and time-consuming method of hair removal which usually concentrates on a small area of hair at a time. A fine needle is inserted into the opening of each hair follicle and a low electric current is passed through the needle to destroy the germinative hair cells, also preventing any new hairs growing from this particular hair follicle. Electrolysis should always be carried out by a qualified professional. It is good for small patches of skin, such as the upper lip and bikini line.

EPILJET

This new treatment takes a full six months but it promises to get rid of unwanted hair permanently and painlessly after 12–16 applications. Unlike

WHICH METHOD OF HAIR REMOVAL IS BEST?

Area to be treated	Best method of removal
underarms	shaving, depilatory creams
forearms	bleaching
nipples	tweezing, electrolysis, Epiljet
bikini line	depilatory creams, sugaring, waxing, Epiljet
legs	sugaring, waxing, shaving, Epiljet

electrolysis, the salon-based treatment can treat a wide area of the body at any one time, and, as a result, is proving particularly popular with transvestites. The treatment involves the application of a vegetable-based gel to the body which is then warmed by bands of infra-red. After 20 minutes the hair is removed. You may not be able to remove all unwanted hair in time for this summer's holiday, but if you start now, next year should be hair-free. Although the treatment is painless and can be used on any part of the body, once the hairs are destroyed they have to be removed by a conventional method of hair removal, such as waxing. For details see Useful Addresses.

SHAVING

Seventy percent of British women prefer wet shaving to other forms of hair removal, and razor manufacturers have at last become fully aware of this fact by creating razors especially designed to cope with a woman's curves. Wet shaving is quick and inexpensive and it gives a much closer shave than electric razors. Each hair is cut off at the surface of the skin and the hair will begin to grow and show again in a couple of days. Shaving is certainly the easiest method of hair removal, but some women find that it makes their hair grow back coarser. Most women will shave their underarms and legs, but prefer not to shave their pubic hair, through fear of nicks and cuts.

SUGARING

This technique was developed by the ancient Egyptians and, like waxing it pulls the hairs out by the roots. It is called sugaring because a mixture of sugar, water, lemon juice and oil is applied to the skin. Then strips of cotton are pressed over this sticky mixture and these are swiftly pulled off taking all hairs with them. Sugaring kits are available from chemists and it is a simple, but messy and time-consuming process to carry out at home. Alternatively, a number of salons and visiting beauty therapists offer sugaring. It tends to be less painful than waxing as the sugar substance sticks to the hair and not to the skin, so there is less pull. Another one of the pros of sugaring is that it is water soluble and any residue left on the skin is easily removed with water.

TWEEZING

Stray hairs which have escaped other methods of hair removal or the few hairs that you may find on your nipples or toes can be best removed with tweezers. This is also the best way to remove hairs from your eyebrows. Tweezing pulls hairs from the roots and it does hurt. A toner or dabs of witch hazel should be applied after plucking to close pores and guard against infection

WAXING

With waxing the hairs are pulled out at the root and the results can last up to six weeks. With continued treatment, regrowth is weakened and the hairs that grow back are softer and less noticeable. You need to have around three weeks' growth before you can have this treatment, whether at home or in a salon. Some women find waxing too painful although it is less so when carried out by a professional. If you have waxing treatments throughout the year it can be quite expensive, but then you are saving on the razor blades! There are three kinds of wax: hot, cold and strip. Hot wax is applied in patches on hairy skin and allowed to cool before being ripped off. Cool wax tends to be slightly gentler than hot wax. For home use, wax-coated strips can be bought from chemists which you simply press on and pull off. These are not always effective.

Each method of hair removal suits a particular area of the body (see table).

SUNCARE

Once you have achieved your smooth, slim figure and are ready to expose your hairless body on the beach or by the pool there is another major consideration if you want to keep your skin looking good – suncare. If you do not protect your skin with sunscreens then you will soon be the colour of a lobster and the pain of sunburn will ruin your summer. The sun's rays can permanently damage our skin by causing premature ageing. Skin cancer is also on the increase with 40,000 new cases being diagnosed in Britain every year. We need to protect ourselves against both ultraviolet A and B rays if we want to stop our skin burning and ageing too quickly. UVB rays are by far the most damaging, being mostly responsible for skin cancer. These rays are absorbed by the epidermis and the upper layers of the dermis, stimulating the production of the pigment melanin which gives us our tan; UVB rays also help us to produce vitamin D in the body. If your skin is exposed to UVB rays for too long it will redden and burn. UVB rays are present whenever the sun shines and are four times stronger in the summer than the winter, between the hours of 11am and 3pm. This is why we should stay out of the midday sun. However, the thinning of the ozone layer means that more UVB rays are now getting through.

UVA rays make up 80 percent of ultraviolet radiation and the damage they cause is less apparent. These rays penetrate deep into the skin's dermis and over time they damage the collagen and elastin fibres which give skin its support, leading to what dermatologists call photo-ageing, or wrinkling. UVA rays are responsible for sun-induced allergies (such as prickly heat) and help generate harmful free-radicals, unstable particles that damage cells. UVA rays are present all year round, even in cloudy weather, which is why you should always wear sun protection. UVA rays are also emitted from sunbeds so, while most tanning machines won't burn, they will accelerate the ageing process within the skin.

SUNSCREENS

Wearing sunscreens means that you can stay in the sun longer and build up your tan steadily while protecting your skin against the damaging effects of UV rays. The safest forms of sunscreen are reflective barriers, such as finely ground titanium dioxide. This simple substance bounces the sun's rays off the skin. When it comes to choosing a sunscreen, the scientific terms can be confusing. The first thing you'll notice on the bottle is the letters 'SPF' (sun protection factor) followed by a number. An SPF is there to tell you how long you can safely stay in the sun without burning; for example, if your bare skin normally reddens after ten minutes in the sun, using a product with SPF8 will allow you to stay out for eighty minutes without burning (10 x 8 = 80). But this will vary from person to person – the paler your skin, the quicker you will burn and the higher the SPF protection you will need to be safe.

Which SPF do I need?

Skin can be divided into six groups, with group one being the fairest and six the darkest. To work out which SPF you need, first decide which skin type you are:

* **Type 1:** Your skin is naturally very pale, with a fine texture and a translucent quality. It freckles easily and always burns in strong sun. It probably reddens within ten minutes of unprotected exposure to sunlight. Your skin never develops a proper tan, and peels after burning. People with this skin type often have fair or red hair and blue or green eyes.

SUN PROTECTION FACTOR CHART

	SPFs for skin type					
	1	2	3	4	5	6
UK/North Europe	10–15	10–12	8–10	6–8	6	4–6
Mediterranean	15–20	12–15	10–12	8–10	6–8	6
Tropics/Africa	20–30	15–25	12–20	10–15	8–10	6–8

* **Type 2:** Your skin is naturally fair and tends to freckle. When exposed to strong sun you burn in about twenty minutes. Your skin does tan, but with difficulty. This is probably the most common skin type in the UK, with most having fair hair and blue eyes.

* **Type 3:** Your skin is medium toned, not really olive but not fair either. You don't usually freckle and your skin tans fairly easily and doesn't usually burn. Your hair is generally dark and your eyes brown.

* **Type 4:** Your skin is olive in tone – the typical Mediterranean look. It doesn't freckle, tans easily and doesn't often burn. But don't be fooled into thinking it doesn't need protection – the ageing UVA rays still penetrate deep into the dermis if you don't protect it. Hair is usually dark and eyes brown.

* **Type 5:** Your skin is naturally brown, typically Asian, Indian, North African or Arabic in origin. Your skin almost never burns and darkens quickly on exposure to sun. Some sun protection is still recommended to guard against wrinkling.

* **Type 6:** Yours is the darkest skin tone, dark brown or black, typically African or West Indian in origin. You never burn and skin darkens quickly on sun exposure. Dermatologists still recommend you protect your skin in strong sunlight.

The level of protection your skin needs will depend on the time of year, which part of the world you are in, and how long you spend outside. Check the SPF table to see which SPF you need.

Written in the stars

Always choose a sunscreen that offers UVA as well as UVB protection. To check the level of UVA screening in a product, Boots has introduced a star rating system which is now featured on major suncare brands. Look at the back of the pack where you will see a number of stars, ranging from one to four. These stars tell you how much UVA protection there is in relation to the UVB protection given. Levels range from one star (minimum) to four stars (maximum). However, these symbols only represent a ratio – an SPF15 product may only have one star, but it will give more protection against UVA rays than an SPF4 product with four stars. It is confusing but, to be safe, opt for a product with a high factor with maximum star rating.

MODERATE

GOOD

SUPERIOR

MAXIMUM

FAKE TAN

One of the worries about wearing a bikini is exposing an ultra-white body, so it is a good idea to use a fake tan to give your skin a bit of colour. Many of us make the mistake of over-exposing our bodies on the first day of the holiday so that we become tanned as quickly as possible. Unfortunately, more often than not, this results in our skin burning, defeating the object as the next couple of days have to be spent in the shade while our skin repairs itself. There are a huge range of self-tanning products available that work in a variety of ways. You can either use waterproof body make-up to tan your skin which can be scrubbed off at the end of the day, or choose a longer-lasting tanning product that contains special tanning agents. The majority of self-tanning products contain dihydroxyacetone (DHA), which binds with the proteins in the skin's surface cells, initially appearing colourless, but gradually turning brown in two to four hours. The tanned effect lasts a few days, until the surface layer of skin is removed. It is important to remember that the majority of tanning products do not protect your skin from the sun so you will still need to apply a sunscreen. Check the self-tanning product first to see if it contains sunscreens. Some manufacturers produce tinted sunscreens so that you can protect your skin from the start and still give your skin the appearance of already being tanned.

AFTER-SUN CARE

The sun has a drying effect on our skin and whether your skin becomes burned or not, it is a good idea to moisturise it when you come in from the sun with a rich after-sun lotion. These creams and lotions usually contain natural ingredients such as cocoa butter, shea butter and aloe vera and they help to cool and soothe our skin. Some after-sun lotions also include skin-saving nutrients such as vitamin E to help repair burnt and damaged skin. Using a massage oil made from soothing essential oils, such as lavender, will also help to restore your skin after a long day in the sun. Here is my recipe for an effective after-sun skin soother.

After-sun skin soother

This semi-solid lotion is excellent for treating mild sunburn, preventing peeling and for prolonging a suntan. It is also deeply remoisturising and can be used as an intensive skin conditioner on areas of parched skin.

25ml (1oz) cocoa butter
30ml (2tbsp) almond oil
15ml (1tbsp) olive oil
5ml (1tsp) wheatgerm oil
10 drops lavender essential oil

Melt the cocoa butter in a small saucepan over a low heat. Add the almond, olive and wheatgerm oils and stir vigorously to mix. Allow to cool and add the lavender essential oil. Pour the mixture into a screw-top bottle or jar.

EXERCISE EXTRAS

We were not designed to lead static lives, where the only movement we make is from the house to the car, and from the car to a chair in the office or a friend's sofa. This daily lack of physical activity will eventually lead to sluggish circulation, poor lymphatic drainage and ill-health. The less exercise we have, the more likely we are to feel tired and run down and inclined to find solace in eating chocolate and other comfort foods. Exercise on its own will not enable us lose weight but it is essential if we wish to tone and firm our bodies and get rid of those extra flabby bits for good!

WHICH EXERCISE?

Aerobic exercise is needed to work our cardiovascular system and get our blood pumping. Regular aerobic exercise will transform us into fitter, leaner people as it not only improves the performance of our heart and lungs, but also burns up excess fat and calories. When we exercise our blood sends extra supplies of nutrients to all our cells, including those in the sluggish tissue of the hips and thighs, and it removes stagnant wastes simultaneously. Our cells are stimulated to release fatty acids and turn them into energy, helping to reduce the size of our thighs and hips. Rates of energy burned for different types of aerobic exercise are listed in the table.

Aerobic exercise does not refer to aerobic classes alone – although this is a sure and fast way to burn up those excess calories. Aerobic exercise is also a good mental stimulus as it produces substances called endorphins which are similar to the drug morphine. These help to relieve any pain as well as giving us a natural high. When aerobics became such a popular form of exercise in the early eighties, many women actually became addicted to it and were doing as many as two or more classes a day. Although aerobic exercise stimulates the

CALORIE COUNTER

Exercise	Approx. Kcals per hour
Step aerobics	600
Skipping	600
Aerobics	550
Swimming	500
Tennis	450
Cycling	400
Badminton	350
Fast walking	300

body in so many different ways, this does not mean that doing it excessively is good for you. Aerobics, in particular, puts a great deal of pressure on the joints and should not be done more than three times a week for more than an hour each time, unless under supervision.

There are many other forms of aerobic exercise which are not quite as demanding as aerobics itself, such as cycling, jogging, swimming or even just walking.

In order to maximise the benefits of exercise, you need to aim to exercise for twenty minutes or more, at 60 percent of your maximum heart rate (MHR), at least three times a week.

First take your pulse by pressing down on the artery at the wrist with three fingers and counting the number of heartbeats that occur over six seconds. Then multiply this figure by ten to calculate your resting heart rate. To work out your maximum heart rate (MHR), subtract your age from 220. Multiply this figure by 0.6 (or by 60 percent), and you will have your target heart rate (THR).

So, if you are thirty years' old:

MHR = 220 – 30 = 190 beats per minute (BPM)
THR = 190BPM x 0.6 = 114BPM

The figure gives you an at a glance guide to your target heart rate (THR).

Choose from the list below to find out which form of aerobic exercise is best suited to you and your lifestyle:

Aerobics – it is best to choose low-impact aerobics rather than the high-impact variety as this is more gentle on your joints, especially if you have not done it before. Almost every health club or sports centre runs aerobic classes and the fact that everything is organised for you is more of an incentive to go on a regular basis. You can also follow one of Mr Motivator's excellent videos in the comfort of your own home. Before you embark on any aerobic exercise it is vitally important that you carry out stretching and warming-up exercises first as these prepare your body for what is in store. If you are suffering from any medical condition which may be affected by exercising, such as back problems, then you should consult your doctor first.

TARGET HEART RATE

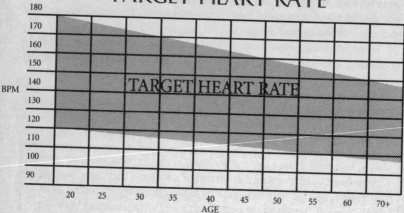

Cycling – this is an excellent form of aerobic exercise which is not tough on your joints, and it will greatly tone your legs. Cycling is also a great form of transport, but not when it is done on busy, main roads where not only do you have to stop and start all the time, but you are also breathing in toxic fumes from cars and diesel lorries. Nowadays, of course, you can cycle in the comfort of your own home on static exercise bikes.

Dancing – exercise does not have to be a repetitive routine of the same short movements, it can also be in the form of something creative such as dance. Dancing, whether it be disco or ballet, may be something which you enjoy doing already for its own sake. So, if you have a busy night life, it is no excuse for not doing any exercise, as the dance floor is the ideal place for some serious blood pumping.

Jogging and running – these two types of exercise really get the blood surging! But they are not suitable for those who have problems with their weight-bearing joints such as knees or ankles. You should avoid running or jogging on concrete pavements or other hard ground as this puts even greater pressure on your joints. Make sure that you wear proper running shoes which provide adequate support and cushioning. If there is a field or park near you then use this, as grass has a certain amount of 'give' which is ideal for this type of aerobic exercise.

Walking – even this everyday activity is aerobic if you put enough energy into it. Either on your way to work or in your lunch hour, you should spend at least ten solid minutes each day walking briskly. To get the best from walking, your back should be straight, tummy held in and, as you walk, sway your hips subtly to either side while swinging your arms. This walk may sound like the 'Ministry of Silly Walks' from

Monty Python's Flying Circus, but it actually looks good. Walking this way not only encourages excellent posture, it also exercises your bottom, thighs and arms and the more movement involved in your walk, the more aerobic it is and the more calories you will burn. As with all other exercises, it is best to walk in fresh air and not beside a busy road, to ensure that you inhale large amounts of oxygen and few toxic fumes.

Rebounding – rebounding on a mini trampoline (or bouncer) is another great form of aerobic exercise and it is believed by some to be the best possible form of exercise for combating cellulite due to the use it makes of the force of gravity. The up-and-down movement, which first suspends your body in space and then subjects it to two or three times the force of gravity, stimulates the elimination of wastes through your lymph system. Increased oxygen is also brought to the cells, boosting the whole system and encouraging general detoxification. Rebounding is something that you can do in the privacy of your own home irrespective of your age, your level of fitness or the weather outside. You can bounce to music or in front of GMTV as a great start to the day (you can even skip at the same time). Another benefit is that you will never be troubled by constipation while you are regularly rebounding.

Swimming – this is a great exercise for toning your whole body and it does not have the problems which weight-bearing exercises have. Even those who have weak ankles, knees or backs can swim, as your body becomes weightless in water and so removes any pressure on these areas. When swimming, you are exercising virtually every major muscle in your body but the water keeps you cool. To get the best out of swimming, you need to swim straight lengths without stopping to rest, for at least twenty minutes. If this is your only exercise, try and do it three times a week, every other day. You could also slip in a few underwater hip and thigh toning exercises at the end of your swimming session. Any exercise you do underwater involves a great deal more effort than on land as the weight of the water restricts your movements.

Here is a complete water workout:

* **For the bottom:** Stand sideways to the pool wall and hold on to the side with one hand. Keeping your back straight and your left foot flat on the pool floor, lift and bend your right knee towards your chest. Straighten your leg out in front of you. Slowly swing the straight leg backwards until you feel your buttocks 'squeeze'. Repeat five–ten times on each leg.

* **For the inner and outer thighs:** Stand sideways to the pool wall and lift the outer leg out to the side as far as possible. Sweep the leg forwards so that it crosses in front of the supporting leg. Sweep the leg out again. Repeat the movement, swinging the leg backwards. Repeat five–ten times on each leg.
* **Finish up** by striding as far as you can up the pool and back again, using your arms to help propel you.

TONING EXERCISES

As well as doing some form of aerobic exercise three times a week, here are some simple toning exercises which concentrate on specific problem areas such as the tummy, bottom, thighs and upper arms. The ten toning exercises outlined here only take ten minutes in all and for the best results you should do them every day in addition to your aerobic activity.

Sit-ups – lie on your back with hands touching your ears and legs slightly apart and bent as shown. Hold your tummy muscles in to protect your back. Raise your head and shoulders slowly off the ground until you can feel the 'crunch' in your stomach muscles then slowly return to the starting position. Complete twenty of these sit-ups. With this exercise you should breathe out as you sit up and breathe in as you sit down.

Diagonal curls – lie on your back with knees bent and lower back flat on the floor. Hold your tummy muscles in to protect your back. With your right hand touching your right ear and right elbow on the floor, raise your head and both shoulders off the floor and bring your left arm over to touch the outside of your right knee. Slowly return to your starting position and continue until you have completed ten of these diagonal curls. Then swap arms so that you are bringing your right arm up and over to touch your left leg. Complete ten more diagonal curls. With this exercise you should breathe out as you curl up and breathe in as you curl down.

Stomach crunches – lie on your back with hands touching your ears, cross your ankles and raise your feet in the air. Tighten the abdominal muscles. Keeping your legs still, raise head and neck off the floor and touch one knee with the opposite elbow. Then return to starting position. Try to get both shoulders off the floor. Complete ten of these movements and then repeat with the other knee and elbow. With this exercise you should breathe out as you curl up and breathe in as you curl down.

Bottoms up – lie on the floor, arms at your sides, knees bent and feet shoulder width apart. Clench your buttocks, tuck in your tummy and raise your pelvis up transferring your weight onto the shoulders (not the legs). Hold for five seconds, relax and repeat ten times.

Bottom and leg lifts – kneel with upper body weight supported on forearms. Keeping your tummy tucked in, straighten your right leg and bring it in line with your back. Keeping your foot flexed, raise your right leg a couple of inches and lower it again. Repeat ten times. Then bend your knee and again move your leg up and down a few inches ten times. Repeat with other leg.

Back thigh lifts – lie on your stomach and rest your head on folded hands. Keeping your head and your hands firmly on the ground, lift both legs up. With your feet flexed kick out to the sides and then bring your feet back together again. Repeat eight times but stop if you feel that it is straining your back.

Then raise one leg at the time, hold for as long as possible and relax back on to the floor. Repeat eight times for each leg as before.

Front of thigh – place your back against a wall and your feet 60cm in front, shoulder width apart. Rest your hands on your legs and slowly lower your back down the wall until your thighs are parallel to the floor. Hold this position for as long as you can – aim for about twenty seconds to start with, gradually building up to a full minute.

Inner thigh – lie flat on the floor, place a cushion between your thighs and raise them up over your stomach. Then squeeze your thighs around the cushion and hold for five seconds, then relax and repeat twenty times to start with, increasing gradually up to fifty repetitions.

Outer thigh – lie on your side supporting your head with your hand and your other hand flat on the floor. Flex your foot and raise your leg slowly up to a height of about 30cm. Lower your leg slowly, but do not touch the floor, and then continue to raise it and lower it until you have completed the exercise ten times. Relax and then raise and lower the leg again – this time pointing and flexing your toes alternatively eight times. Repeat the whole exercise with the other leg.

Arm twirls – stand up straight with your arms outstretched on either side. Simply move your arms forwards in a circular motion ten times. Then move them back the other way ten times. If you feel that you can, repeat and vary the size of the circular movement.

Elbow presses – stand up straight with your arms outstretched. Bend your arms at the elbow as shown and bring both arms in front of you so that they meet. Pull your arms back again to the starting position and repeat sixteen times. On the last time that your arms are bought together, hold the position and move them up and down together a small distance. Repeat sixteen times.

EFFORTLESS EXERCISE - SALON TREATMENTS

Electrotherapy

There are a number of fat-burning, tummy-toning, cellulite-busting salon treatments available throughout the UK, many of which involve electrotherapy. This technology was first used by physiotherapists to 're-educate' the muscles of those involved in accidents who could no longer move a certain part of their body so that their muscles would not waste away. It was also used for those who had experienced paralysis due to strokes and for those with Bell's Palsy where certain muscles in the face are paralysed. Electrotherapy has recently been adopted by the slimming industry with some dramatic results in terms of inch-loss and combating cellulite. Electrotherapy exercises our muscle and skin tissue by sending minute electronic impulses through our skin to the underlying muscle. There are a wide variety of these treatments available all using slightly different microcurrents of electricity.

One of the most well-known treatments is the Face and Body Perfector where the flow of current is applied to the skin via two hand-held cotton-tipped electrodes, to stimulate a specific area such as the thighs or the stomach. Unfortunately, it can only be used on one area of the body at a time, but it is a good way of tightening flabby arms, slack tummies and bulging hips and thighs. It is also ideal for tightening loose skin caused by considerable weight-loss and is said to help reduce cellulite by encouraging the lymphatic drainage system to remove toxins from the body, while speeding the dispersal of fat deposits. It also claims to reduce and improve the appearance of stretchmarks significantly if they are treated early enough. Stretchmarks show up particularly in summer as they do not tan with the rest of the body. The Face and Body Perfector is currently available in over 140 salons nationwide and treatment for each part of the body costs around £15 for a half-hour session (see Useful Addresses).

Electronic Inch-Loss

One of the most recently developed inch-loss systems is Arasys which also uses electronic currents to tone muscle tissue. The current is in the form of a unique faradic wave that hits a wide area of the muscle and, therefore, minimises pain. The first electronic inch-loss systems were fairly painful as the wave shape of the current meant that it would hit the muscle in full force at a tiny point. Thankfully, the Arasys system is pain-free, although it does take a bit of getting used to. Damp pads containing metal plates are placed over the areas of the body that are being worked on and these are held firmly in place with rubber bands. The current is applied through wires connecting the pads to the electronically programmed Arasys machine. The thought of damp pads and electricity may set alarm bells ringing, but it is perfectly safe. One of the main benefits of Arasys is that it can be used to tone many different parts of the body simultaneously. For most of us, this will mean the buttocks, tummy, outer thighs and inner thighs. Each session lasts for seventeen minutes and the current is applied in doses lasting a few seconds. At first, the intensity of the current is very mild and creates a slight tingling sensation. It is then increased throughout the session so that the muscle contractions are much more powerful. It is a very odd sensation lying down and feeling and seeing your muscles contract and relax without having any control over it. If you hate exercise, or unable to workout, then this is one effortless way to achieve great muscle tone – one Arasys session is said to equal two to three hours in the gym or 300 sit-ups! Arasys is currently available at around seventy salons nationwide and each session costs about £15, with special deals for courses (see Useful Addresses).

Toning tables

These are another way of exercising your muscles effortlessly. There are different tables for exercising different muscles: one for your legs, one for your stomach, one for your hips, etc. All you have to do is lie back as the table lifts and stretches various parts of your body without you having to do a thing. A client usually spends about ten minutes on each table which adds up to the equivalent of a two-mile walk, 900 back-kicks and ninety sit-ups! Toning tables are found in many beauty salons nationwide.

Please note: Electrotherapy treatments and toning tables do not exercise our cardiovascular system at all. They work on our muscles alone and aerobic exercise is required to stimulate our circulation and the heart – the most important muscle of all!

AND FINALLY ... HOW TO CHOOSE YOUR BIKINI!

Finding the perfect swimming costume or bikini for the summer can be difficult and often stressful, but selecting the right cut, pattern and colour to suit your particular body shape and skin tone is vital for looking good on the beach or by the pool. Not everybody ends up with a perfect figure even after successful weight-loss, but following a few fashion pointers can really make a difference. A swimsuit sagging in the swimming pool or one which suddenly turns transparent on contact with water are just two of the nightmares we can avoid.

Fortunately the larger stores are trying to make this annual task easier. Some produce brochures giving guidelines on the various styles available and those most suitable for your particular shape, others are offering a 'pick 'n' mix' option which allows us to buy different sizes of bikini top and bottom, if necessary. In addition there are several new interesting inventions, including a 'tan-through' fabric which could mean an end to strap marks. The Janet Frazer catalogue offers a 'design your own bikini' service which allows freedom of choosing two bikini tops (one for sun-bathing, one for swimming) to go with one matching bottom. Lands End is another mail-order service with fashionable, well-cut bikinis. (See Useful Addresses.)

MEASURING UP

Before you order your swimwear from a catalogue or hit the shops make sure you have an accurate note of your measurements. Don't rely on guesswork unless you want to end up with a swimsuit or bikini that either sags unflatteringly or cuts into your skin.

Bust   measure around your fullest part, keeping the tape measure straight at the back.

Waist bend to one side to find its natural crease. Then standing straight, make sure the tape measure fits comfortably around you.

Hips   measure at their fullest point, making sure the tape is straight and parallel to the floor.

THE CUT

This is perhaps the most important, single element to consider. Although you will now be many pounds lighter than a few weeks ago we all have different body shapes from one another so it is important to be aware of which swimming costume or bikini will suit you best. Apart from the obvious dilemma between the high- or low-cut leg, there are many other options to take into consideration. For example, Speedo has a range of *twelve* different backs!

There are several little tricks which are vital when wanting to enhance a flatter chest or reduce a larger one. This year there is good news for those with a long torso, whose problem in the past has been one of unsightly shoulder straps digging in, as many shops now have a longer body length available. Even better news for those who may have strayed from the *Bikini Diet* – is the Slim Suit or Miracle Suit. It claims to enable us to 'lose 10lb in ten minutes' and it works by having double-strength lycra to hold the stomach in. No need to worry about those poolside lunches if you want a temporary weight-loss effect.

It is widely thought that a high-cut leg will give a longer leg effect, but if care is not given to the pattern this can draw attention to the hip area. It also needs quite a lot of courage to step out on the first morning, when the perfect tan has not yet been achieved. After all, this may be the most revealing item you will wear all year. The lower leg is often popular with the more conservative, giving a longer body effect and a classic, almost Fifties glamour style. The 'boy-line' leg which comes down to the top of the thigh has not been popular despite its fashionable status. It is not very flattering, unless you are lucky enough to have a slim, athletic (and totally cellulite-free) figure.

less revealing covering scars, etc

panels reducing hips

curves accentuate 'hourglass' figure

colour panelling (darker colours produces a slimmer effect)

black

no straps, ideal for sunbathing

more support for smaller chests

bust support

fashionable style but only flattering for the more athletic figure

silhouette panelling

material panelling, attention to seams

The overall trend this year is for bikini bra-style tops with matching hipster shorts or shorts with little belts. If you are feeling brave enough to wear any of these styles, you really need a firm tum, as they draw attention to this area.

ATTENTION TO DETAIL

The use of coloured panels and attention to seams is flattering for the more rounded figure, at the same time offering more support. This follows a move to a corsetry and lingerie look in swimwear, which can increase confidence when the costume is used for more than just sunbathing. The use of panels can also enhance the curves on a flatter figure, especially if the panels are in a patterned material against a darker plain-coloured background. Basically, the more detail to seams or panelling the swimsuit has, the more flexible and versatile it will be, such as being used as a top under a shirt or simply with a pair of beach shorts.

Following the huge success of the Wonderbra, the trend continues towards underwired and padded swimwear. Some stores now offer specific bra sizes (Triumph have a range of DD and E cups available). Padded and moulded cups will also help you achieve the cleavage you want. BhS moulded swimwear cups are designed never to collapse and, as well as offering support for the larger bosom, can also enhance the flatter chest. Underwiring can boost confidence by increasing support and also makes the swimming costume more versatile – it can be worn as a body both in the daytime and during the evening, especially as many shops offer a range a matching co-ordinates such as wraps, shirts and trousers.

For the more sporting look, support and structure is given by panelling the swimming costume, although it may not be underwired. Alternatively, seams around the bosom and material gathered in at the centre can enhance and support without the rigidity of actual underwiring. A more covering style, which may cover the chest entirely up to the neck, is stylish and popular with women who have had a mastectomy or other breast operation.

MATERIAL WORLD

Following the main fashion themes, the fabric looks continue to be glamorous for swimwear this year. There is a trend towards glossy lycras, with many stores offering a super-sexy 'wet-look' range. However, cotton lycra is still very popular for those who prefer a more natural fibre next to their skin. Seersucker is always a popular choice, especially in pretty gingham checks. But be careful! If the material is thick it can give the illusion of adding those pounds you've just lost.

Perhaps the most exciting news as far as material goes is the brand new Sun Select fabric from Triumph. Unbelievably, this allows us to tan through our swimming costume. It's been designed to block harmful UVB rays, only allowing the safer UVA rays through the costume to the skin. Of course, you should still wear protective sun cream under your costume to prevent burning and skin ageing. (Make sure that your suncream has UVA protection as well as UVB protection as it is these rays which penetrate deep into the skin, causing premature ageing.) Triumph have also developed another new material, which is quick drying – handy for swimming holidays. It is a mixture of nylon and lycra with a layer of Teflon which makes water literally roll off the surface like on a non-stick pan. This could be handy if the weather isn't as good as promised – you won't have to drip dry.

COLOUR

Once you've decided the shape and fabric to go for, consider the colour. This has an important effect on the final look. Many women take two swimsuits on holidays, one to suit a paler skin tone and one for when the perfect light tan has been achieved. Bright fluorescent colours contrast brilliantly with a tanned skin, but for a paler skin tone the more classic colours, such as navy, white and black are more flattering. Chocolate browns, beiges and animal prints are also very popular at the moment and look out for the blocks of colour and patterns around the hip area which can give a slimming effect. The use of cleverly patterned panels over the hip area can give a slimming effect. A basic rule to follow is that if you want to reduce your size further, go for smaller patterns. The traditional idea of vertical stripes and darker colours for the larger woman still works well and can be improved by a good use of panels which draw the eye to certain areas, taking attention away from others. On the other hand, those who want to create the illusion of a larger bust, for example, should choose a brightly shaded material with a larger pattern.

BIKINIS

As with swimming costumes, bikinis come in a wide variety of cuts to cater for our different body shapes. The string bikini may be fashionable, but it is extremely revealing! Even supermodels with tiny bottoms and thighs struggle to look good in these. If you don't fancy baring all on the beach, opt for a less revealing cut. A top tip is to choose a highwaisted bikini bottom as it helps to hide a not-too-flat stomach. Again, following high street fashion, the cleavage is big news. Many stores have incorporated this into the bikini, including Wonderbra themselves. The bonus with this type of bikini is that they come in different bra cup sizes, and not just the all-encompassing sizes 10, 12, etc.

Some of the more popular styles are shown in the illustration, where the sporty look is evident in the cropped tops. This top has the advantage of being more concealing, and supportive for all exercise including swimming, although

string bikini – fortunately not too fashionable this year; can be very hard to wear

no straps – good for sunbathing but watch out in the pool!

underwired

wonderbra bikini good for smaller busts

high waistband, flattering 'sporty' style

underwired for support

cropped top

underwired and rippled to enhance the smaller bust

halterneck offers greater security

more concealing 'sporty' look

the straps can cause unsightly white marks and uneven tanning. The strapless top is still a favourite for sunbathing, and on some designs optional halterneck straps allow more security when taking the plunge into the pool.

ACCESSORIES

Matching wraps (called pareos or sarongs), shirts, skirts and even trousers are increasingly on offer, making the bikini even more versatile and holiday packing easier. Choosing a bikini that offers more support on top means that it can be worn away from the beach as well as for simply soaking up the sun.

There is now a much wider choice as the distinction between swimwear and casual wear blurs, and finding a swimsuit with a perfect fit is getting easier. The bikini itself is moving away from the sea front and poolside and on to the streets. With your new slimline shape it can carry you through the day with confidence and style.

USEFUL ADDRESSES

PRODUCE SUPPLIERS

Barleycorn: 97–99 Lancaster Road, Enfield EN2 0JN. Tel: 0181-363 2345 Fax: 0181-364 4266. Extensive selection of health foods and organic fruits and vegetables. Regular delivery service throughout Greater London. Catalogue available.

Freshlands: 196 Old Street, London EC1V 9FR. Tel: 0171 490 3170. Extensive mail-order selection of foods, including unusual oriental ingredients, cookware and books. Catalogue available.

Randalls Butchers: 113 Wandsworth Bridge Road, London SW6. Tel: 0171-736 3426. The best butcher in London for free-range and organic meat.

Rubicon Health: Second Way, Wembley, Middx. HA9. Tel: 0181 900 9944. Importers of low-fat coconut water. Contact direct for local stockists.

The Watermill: Little Salkeld, Penrith CA10 1NN. Tel: 01768 881523. Mail-order suppliers of organic stoneground flours. Will also despatch organic cereals, wholegrains, dried fruits, nuts, seeds and herb teas. Catalogue available.

Whole Earth Foods Ltd: 269 Portobello Road, London W11 1LR. Tel: 0171-229 7545 Manufacturers of health foods including precooked tinned brown rice. Send an SAE for a free natural food guide and stockists.

Wholefood: 24 Paddington Street, London W1M 4DR. Tel: 0171-935 3924. The first health-food shop to supply a wide range of organic produce. Also stocks an extensive selection of foods and supplements, plus books and journals on health, nutrition and organic gardening. Mail-order service available.

BODY BRUSH AND COSMETIC SUPPLIERS

Selected branches of **Boots** and **The Body Shop** or by mail order from:

Green Farm: 225 Putney Bridge Road, London SW15 2PY.
Tel: 0181-874 1130/5631

Dermablend: Gemini House, Flew Meadow, Harlow, Essex CM19 5TJ.
Tel: 01279 421 555

ELECTROTHERAPY SUPPLIERS

Arasys Ltd: 5 Brewer Street, London W1R 3FN. Tel: 0171 734 1885

Face and Body Perfector: 10–12 High Street, Burnham, Bucks SL1 7JH.
Tel: 01628 660123

JUICING EQUIPMENT

Wholistic Research Company: Bright Haven, Robin's Lane, Lolworth, Cambridge CB3 8HH. Tel: 01954 781074. Can supply several different types of juicing equipment and water purifiers. Catalogue available.

SLIMMING AIDS

Fat Magnets: Order and enquiry line. Tel.: 0990 997755

AromaTrim™: Order and enquiry line. Tel.: 0116 274 3000

The Daniello Clinic: 59 Bury Old Sreet, Prestwich, Manchester M25 8FG. Freephone 0800 616658

SUPPORT GROUPS

British Dietetic Association: 7th Floor, Elizabeth House, 22 Suffolk Street, Queensway, Birmingham B1 1LS. Tel: 0121-643 5483

The Coronary Prevention Group: 42 Store Street, London WC1E 7DB. Tel: 0171-580 1070

Health Education Authority: Hamilton House, Mabledon Place, London WC1H 9TX. Tel: 0171-383 3833

London School of Hygiene: Dept of Public Health and Policy, 42 Store Street, London WC1E 7DB

The Institute for Complementary Medicine PO Box 194, London SE16 1QZ. Tel: 0171-237 5165. Contact the Institute for a list of practitioners in your area and details of courses in nutrition and complementary therapies. Enclose an SAE.

The Soil Association: 86 Colston Street, Bristol BS1 5BB. Tel: 0117 929 0661. Their symbol is a consumer guarantee that food is high quality and genuinely organically grown, i.e. without the use of pesticides and fungicides. The Soil Association welcomes new members and can also advise on local stockists of organically grown produce around the country. Send an SAE for a list of farmers and stockists in your area.

Vegetarian Society of the United Kingdom Parkdale, Dunham Road, Altrincham WA14 4QG. Tel: 0161-928 0793

SWIMWEAR STOCKISTS

Bhs: Marylebone House, 129–137 Marylebone Road, London NW1 5QD. Tel: 0171-262 3288

Janet Frazer: Tel: 0345 888 222. Mail-order catalogue available

Land's End: Tel: Freephone 0800 220106. Mail-order catalogue available

Miracle Suit: Similar to Slim Suit. Available exclusively from Harrods, Knightsbridge, London SW1X 7QX (tel: 0171-730 1234). Prices start at £75 up to £120. Assorted styles and colours available.

Slim Suit: *Great Universal Fashion Extra* catalogue. Tel: Freephone 0500 923923. Available in sizes 12, 14, 16 and 18, price around £59.99. Black and white only.

Speedo: Speedo Europe Ltd, Ascot Road, Nottingham NG8 5AJ. Tel: 0115 929 6131. Available from all good sports shops.

Triumph: For your nearest stockists telephone 01793 720330. Triumph swimwear is available at House of Fraser, John Lewis and Selfridges.

RECIPE INDEX

Recipe Index

INDEX

Index

LIZ EARLE'S
NATURAL SKINCARE

For further information about Liz Earle's own range of ethical
skincare made without petro-chemicals but with high levels of
naturally active ingredients such as vitamins and the herb
echinacea, send a large stamped addressed envelope to
Liz Earle
PO Box 11644
London NW6 1LE
United Kingdom
Or telephone Freephone 0800 413318

Liz Earle ethical skincare

No petro-chemicals

No chemical sunscreens

No animal testing

Every purchase supports charities

HOW TO ORDER YOUR BOXTREE BOOKS BY LIZ EARLE

- ☐ 0 7522 0558 7 Aromatherapy — £3.99
- ☐ 0 7522 2100 0 Baby and Toddler Foods — £3.99
- ☐ 1 85283 543 5 Food Facts — £3.99
- ☐ 1 85283 546 X Vegetarian Cookery — £3.99
- ☐ 0 7522 1619 8 Evening Primrose Oil — £3.99
- ☐ 0 7522 1614 7 Herbs for Health — £3.99
- ☐ 1 85283 984 8 Successful Slimming — £3.99
- ☐ 0 7522 9553 6 Vitamins and Minerals — £3.99
- ☐ 0 7522 2105 1 Detox — £3.99
- ☐ 0 7522 1635 X Hair Loss — £3.99
- ☐ 0 7522 0544 7 Youthful Skin — £3.99
- ☐ 0 7522 1680 5 Healthy Pregnancy — £3.99
- ☐ 0 7522 0548 X Dry Skin and Eczema — £3.99
- ☐ 0 7522 1641 4 Cod Liver Oil — £3.99
- ☐ 0 7522 0599 4 Juicing — £3.99
- ☐ 0 7522 1631 7 Acne — £3.99
- ☐ 0 7522 1673 2 Food Combining — £3.99
- ☐ 0 7522 1690 2 Post-natal Health — £3.99
- ☐ 0 7522 1675 9 Food Allergies — £3.99
- ☐ 0 7522 1685 6 Healthy Menopause — £3.99
- ☐ 0 7522 1668 6 Beating PMS — £3.99
- ☐ 0 7522 1663 5 Antioxidants — £3.99
- ☐ 1 85283 518 4 Liz Earle's ACE Plan: The New Guide to Super Vitamins A, C and E — £4.99
- ☐ 1 85283 554 0 Liz Earle's ACE Plan Weight-loss for Life — £4.99

All books shown are available at your local bookshop or can be ordered direct from the publisher. Just tick the titles you want and fill in the form below. Prices and availability subject to change without notice.

Macmillan C.S. Dept, Macmillan Distribution Ltd, Houndmills, Basingstoke RG24 2XS. Or telephone 01256 29242

Please send cheque or postal order for the value of the book(s), and add £1.00 for one book, plus 50p for each additional book, for postage and packing. Applicable only in the UK, and BFPO addresses. Payment may be made in sterling or by UK personal cheque, postal order, sterling draft or international money order, made payable to Pan Books Ltd. Alternatively by VISA/Mastercard/Amex/Diners.

Card number ☐☐☐☐☐☐☐☐☐☐☐☐☐☐☐☐

Amount £ ....

Expiry date on card ....

Signed ....

PLEASE COMPLETE IN BLOCK LETTERS

Name ....

Address ....